Calisthenics:

Stretch Your Way

To

Strong

CALISTHENICS STRETCH YOUR WAY TO STRONG

THE #1 FLEXIBILITY FOR BODYWEIGHT TRAINING GUIDE

PURECALISTHENICS

Disclaimer:

This guide has been created for informational and reference purposes only. The author, publisher and other affiliated parties cannot be held in any way accountable for any personal injuries or damage allegedly resulting from the information contained herein, or from any misuse of such guidance. Although strict measures have been taken to provide accurate information, the parties involved with the creation and publication of this guide take no responsibility for any issues that may arise from alleged discrepancies contained herein. It is strongly recommended that you consult a physician, personal trainer and nutritionist prior to commencing this or any other workout or diet plan. This guide is not a substitute for professional personal guidance from a qualified medical professional. If you feel pain or discomfort at any point during the exercises contained herein, cease the activity immediately and seek medical guidance. This resource has been created to teach stretching in a progressive manner, and you should not advance until you have completed the simpler stretches as recommended with perfect form. It is strongly recommended that you use a spotter or personal trainer at all times.

calisthenics

[kal-*uh* s-**then**-iks]

Noun

1. *Gymnastic exercises designed to develop physical strength, vigor and grace of movement, usually performed with little or no special apparatus.*

Origin

Greek *kallos* "beauty" + *sthenos* "strength" + -ics.

BEFORE YOU BEGIN:

FREE BONUS STRETCHING GUIDE

Stretching wrong can be costly in more ways than one. At best you may simply fail to make any progress towards your flexibility goals, and at worst you may do serious damage to your muscles, ligaments or tendons. Not on our watch!

To avoid injury and help accelerate your progress, pick up our free 'Top 10 Stretching Mistakes' guide to make sure YOU aren't falling into these common traps.

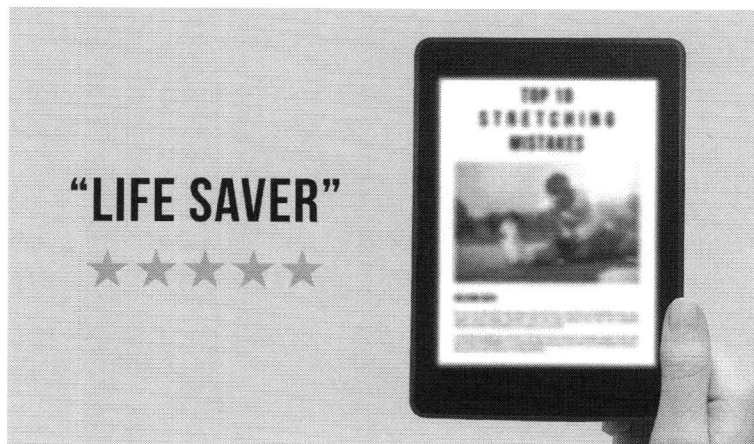

"LIFE SAVER"

★★★★★

Visit www.purecalisthenics.com/stretching-guide to get yours now!

CONTENTS

INTRODUCTION

You have a hidden weakness, a chink in your armor, holding you back from achieving your full potential in calisthenics and bodyweight exercise.

You can't quite hold a certain position; perfect form often evades you and those last few reps are tantalizingly out of reach. You know your body is capable of more, but you just can't level up and as a result your progress plateaus.

Just how the hell do all these YouTube superstars manage to make it all look so damn easy? Well, amigos, they have a secret weapon, and its name is range of motion.

Range of motion is defined as the positions at which you start, move through and finish any particular exercise. Tight muscles = shorter range of motion = less strength.

With greater flexibility, therefore, comes greater range of motion, and with it superior strength building ability. This cycle repeats all the way to SUPERHUMAN!

The bad news is you've probably been stretching wrong all your life. Seriously, even if you are absolutely, positively certain that you know it all, we're willing to bet you're missing something. The good news is, the secret formula is right here in your hands.

Using five simple scientific techniques you will see immediate improvements in both your flexibility and ROM. This, in turn, will allow you to compound your strength and muscle gains at unprecedented rates.

Join us as we dive into the latest installment in The SUPERHUMAN Series and get set to experience mind-blowing results.

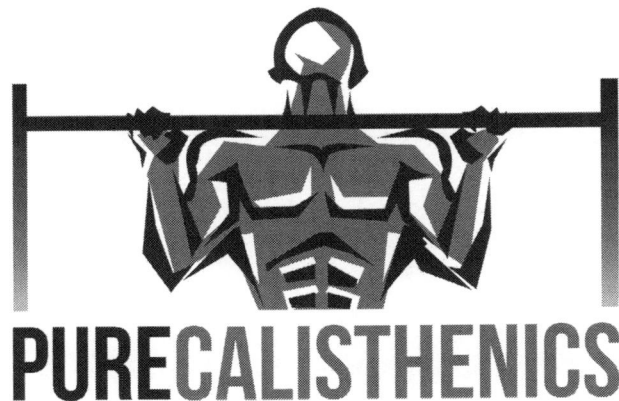

PURECALISTHENICS

1. FLEXIBILITY IN A NUTSHELL

STRETCHING DOES NOT GUARANTEE FLEXIBILITY

You're going to have to get used to the fact that much of what you have been told to date is untrue. So, this eye-opener seems a good place to start.

Of course, stretching *is* a prerequisite for flexibility, but it is only one piece of the puzzle, and while you can make progress through exercises alone, you may find it a slow and frustrating process. But don't worry, you're not alone!

It's a commonly held misconception throughout the fitness community that in order to achieve your desired level of flexibility a rigorous regime of stretching is required to increase elasticity and prevent your muscles from shortening and tightening over time.

We're here to show you a much faster and more sustainable route to success, and we're guaran-damn-teeing results!

THE SCIENCE

When you complete a strenuous exercise, very tiny tears appear in your target muscles. This is due to the intense physical trauma they were just put through, and when they heal they generally increase in both size and performance. However, when the muscle healing process is taking place, a small amount of scar tissue is formed, which has the effect of 'pulling' the muscle fibers together, effectively making it 'shorter' or 'tighter'.

What's more, with age comes degradation of the connective tissues throughout your body. As you get older, your elastin levels slowly decrease. These elastin proteins are the components in your ligaments and tendons that allow them to deform and return to their original shape, or 'flex'. As your elastin levels drop, so does the range of motion that these connective tissues can tolerate.

So how is it that we sometimes come across folks well into their 60s and 70s who are still as supple as a wet noodle?

It is here that some coaches might step in and say that strenuous and perhaps painful stretching is required to counteract the muscle-shortening effect, but if grandmothers and grandfathers across the globe can maintain their flexibility then surely there must be an easier way! To get there we need to think smarter, not harder.

IT'S ALL IN YOUR HEAD

Or, more precisely, your nervous system. Day-to-day we keep our bodies in the same general envelope of movement. We sit in the same posture, walk around with the same motion, and relax in the same pose. This repetitive use of our body creates what can be thought of as the blueprint of how our muscles generally move, and our brain follows that blueprint to the letter.

Make no mistake; your brain is one crotchety, retentive piece of work. No matter how much you may try to force the issue, it will always automatically resist moving your muscles out of its predetermined comfort zone.

To see this in practice for yourself, try this well-known little drill:

1. Take one leg and lift it to the side at 90 degrees, placing it on a chair or table. Pretty easy isn't it? OK, next step.

2. Now lower that leg and repeat with the other. That feels pretty easy too, huh? Let's ramp it up a notch.

3. Prepare to do the splits. What's that? What do you mean you can't?! You've just had each leg at a 90-degree angle individually, so what's stopping you doing both at the same time?

Believe it or not, there are no physical barriers to you completing this exercise. Zip, zilch, nada, and zero.

What you're experiencing is your body's automatic control system taking over. It allows you to move your legs to 90 degrees individually, but when you try to do both at the same time - something completely alien to most people - everything gets locked down.

Your nervous system, then, keeps you confined to your standard range of motion even when it is abundantly clear that your body is capable of more. Pretty frustrating, huh?

Fear not, young grasshopper, you will soon discover exactly how to break through these barriers and achieve astonishing feats of flexibility. The following tutorials have been written for the express purpose of loosening this deeply rooted subconscious control over your muscles, consequently allowing you to build the physique you long for.

Whether you want to conquer the splits or simply increase your range of motion for a specific exercise, our formula will get you there. So, let's get started, shall we?

"**Physical fitness is not only one of the most important keys to a healthy body, it is the basis of dynamic and creative intellectual activity.**"

John F. Kennedy

2. How to Use This Book

This book is your flexibility bible. You should not simply read the words, but *live* by them. Knowledge is nothing without action, and you will need to take serious action if you want to get serious results. Use these 5 quick tips to get the most out of this guide:

1. Know your Body

Think you know your body? Think again! It's one thing to perform a bit of pre-workout stretching every once in a while but it is something else entirely to undertake a serious stretching regime.

Putting your body under strain can be dangerous if you don't know what you are doing, so it is imperative to familiarize yourself with the key areas of your body to ensure you are utilizing our tutorials correctly and not putting yourself at risk of harm.

We've provided a simple body map on the next page, but we strongly recommend that you take your research further. Get on first name terms with all the major muscle groups so you can target them each with laser-like precision.

You can never be too knowledgeable when it comes to your own body, and we fully encourage people to take a personal trainer's approach. Leave nothing to chance and you will be in complete control of your results. If you're not sure where to start, book a consultation with a professional and they will be able to point you in the right direction.

Super important: if at any time you feel pain or discomfort while stretching, STOP! Try some slow, steady movements to test the area and stretch it out gently to see if the discomfort eases or increases.

If pain persists or worsens, call it a day and seek advice on the issue. Refer back to the body map to hone in on the area and speak to a physician for further guidance.

Only return to stretching or training when you can comfortably perform movements without feeling any impingements or pain. There is no glory in powering on through injuries, you might put yourself out for a long time and jeopardize your results to date.

N.B. For the most part we will use informal names for muscles in this guide because, let's face it, we're not all Latin scholars! You will find the medical names of the most commonly mentioned muscles on the diagram overleaf, along with translations.

Sternocleidomastoid
Trapezius

Deltoid
Pectoralis Major
Rectus abdominis
External Oblique
Latissimus dorsi

Triceps brachii
Biceps brachii
Finger flexors
Finger extensors

Gluteus maximus
Sartorius
Adductor longus
Rectus femoris
Semimembranosus
Biceps femoris

Gastrocnemius
Soleus

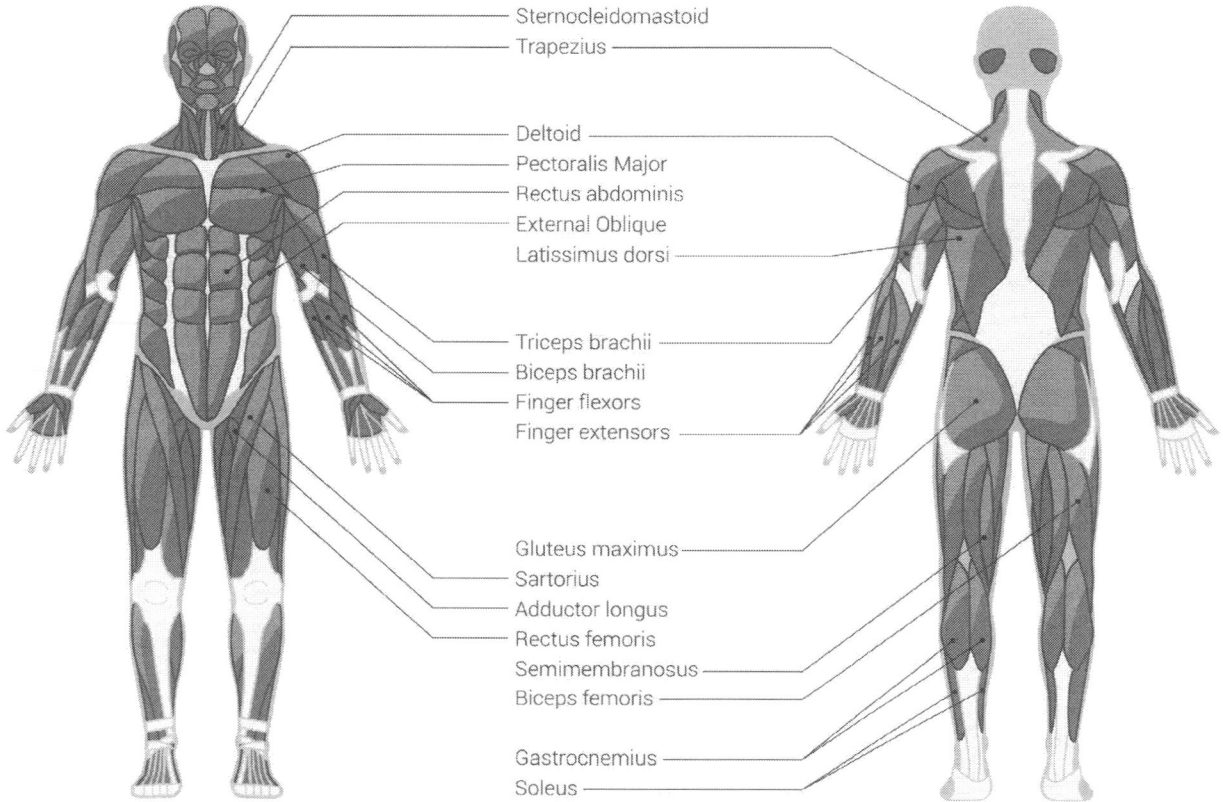

TRANSLATIONS & CONNECTIONS:

Sternocleidomastoid.......Side Neck
Trapezius.......Traps
Deltoid.......Delts
Pectoralis Major.......Pecs / Chest
Rectus Abdominis / External Oblique.......Abs / Obliques
Latissimus Dorsi.......Lats
Triceps Brachii.......Triceps / Tris
Biceps Brachii.......Biceps / Bis
Finger Flexors / Extensors.......Forearms
Gluteus Maximus.......Glutes / Butt!
Sartorius / Adductor Longus.......Hip Flexor
Semimembranosus / Biceps Femoris.......Hamstring
Rectus Femoris.......Quads / Hip Flexor
Gastrocnemius / Soleus.......Calves

2. TRAIN FOR YOUR GOALS

Training for flexibility to help reach your calisthenics goals is not just about physical strength, but mental fortitude, too. Your friends may be chest-bumping freeweight bros who think stretching is for hippies and there's nothing wrong with that. You, however, are training to achieve complete body perfection and you must stand by your decision. Don't allow anyone to influence your thinking – you are training for YOUR goals, not theirs. Live and let live, train and let train!

3. COMMIT

As with any form of exercise you need to be fully committed to a consistent stretching schedule if you want to see results. Don't think you can simply throw in a few here and there and hit the splits in six weeks. Training your nervous system requires dedication. Set a plan and stick to it like glue.

4. BE PATIENT

Following on from the above, it is important to maintain a long-term vision for your stretching. There is no miracle equation for a better body, but flexibility + calisthenics is as close as you can get. Set attainable goals and commit to achieving them within a specific and reasonable time frame. Have faith in the formula, it will get you there!

5. EAT RIGHT & HYDRATE

You may well be forgiven for thinking that dietary advice is relevant exclusively to your calisthenics training program and not your stretching schedule, but the truth is that your body doesn't know the difference between one form of exercise or the other and uses the same fuel to repair and grow regardless of what you put it through.

Your particular goals will determine your diet, but there are some general guidelines to follow here if you want to get in the best shape possible.

Eat clean: We're not asking you to become go plucking fruit from trees, but it really pays to cut out processed food and other junk. Check the labels and pick up fresh foods which contain a single ingredient – i.e. whatever it is actually supposed to be – rather than something packed full of preservatives and lord knows what else.

Mix it up: You've heard it said over and over and now you're going to hear it once again; a balanced and varied diet is the key to good health. This means a mixture of proteins, carbohydrates and fats congruent with your personal goals.

Eat smart: There are plenty of resources out there to assist you with your particular goals and objectives, but we would advise against obsessive calorie counting. Food should be something to look forward to and you will begin to resent it if preparation becomes a chore. By all means use tools and technology to ensure you are on the right track, but don't beat yourself up over fractions of a gram.

With that said, you should be aware of your macros and make a conscious effort to meet them on a daily basis. If you're not sure what this means, it is essentially just the combination of fats, carbs, calories, proteins, etc. which make up your diet. Everybody is different and only you can determine what is appropriate for yourself, but if you are unsure, it pays to contact a professional nutritionist for guidance.

Planning meals in advance and cooking in bulk is super useful here, as it cuts out the guesswork and reduces the risk of making poor decisions on impulse!

We could write a whole book on diet and nutrition, and perhaps we will, but this one is about flexibility, so for now we must move on. Suffice it to say, though, that you should pay special attention to your diet and take the time to investigate it thoroughly in order to maximize your results.

Drink up: Water is life. We need it to transport vital nutrients around the body and to keep our muscles and minds functioning at full capacity.

Most people simply do not drink enough water day-to-day, which means both their performance *and* their recovery is greatly impaired.

According to The European Food Safety Authority, men should be drinking about 2 liters of water per day while women should get about 1.6 liters. This is, of course, a general guideline but if you are not hitting these figures you may be affected by dehydration. We recommend speaking to a physician or nutritionist to discuss your requirements.

That's a wrap on this section. Just remember, you always get out what you put in!

"Patience, persistence and perspiration make an unbeatable combination for success."

Napoleon Hill

3. THE FLEXIBILITY FORMULA

The formula for accomplishing superhuman feats of flexibility consists of three very straightforward principles. First, you need to...

RELAX

If you've tried yoga or the like you may be familiar with being told to 'relaaax' in order to reach the full potential of a pose. This isn't only for the purpose of setting your everyday anxieties aside and enjoying some peace, there's real science at work here.

Your nervous system needs to relax its grip on your muscles in order to make progress in a stretch. As we mentioned earlier, as soon as your brain detects muscle movement outside its expected and predefined blueprint it immediately commands the offending muscles to tighten and prevent further progress.

This lock down effect is the source of all that tension and pain you feel when you push the envelope. To overcome this and redefine your blueprint you must do something completely counterintuitive.

Try telling a pregnant woman to relax during contractions and you'll quite likely get the nearest blunt object hurled at your head with venom. This is an extreme example and we DO NOT recommend trying that at home, but we all face the same battle internally.

It seems a ridiculous suggestion, to relax when your every muscle fiber is screaming otherwise. Thankfully we have a few hacks to override your body's automatic 'freak out' response system and allow your muscles to effortlessly slide to their full potential.

Once you've mastered this fundamental step you must embrace your newfound skill of relaxation to encourage further flexibility, all without pushing your muscles too far, too fast. To achieve this you next need to...

TRAIN

You may soon be able to coax your nervous system into allowing your muscles to begin moving beyond their previous limits, but pushing them to unsafe or damaging levels will cause those barriers to shoot right back up.

For example, let's say the defense system goes offline, you are relaxed and you sink straight into SUPER deep stretch, further than you've ever managed before. What do you suppose is the first thing that will happen? If you are human, it's quite likely that you will suddenly become very much aware of how unfamiliar this new position is, and that will lead to immediate concerns over whether or not it is safe. The second you become even the slightest bit concerned about causing damage, your muscles will tense up and this may result in the very injury you were so desperate to avoid in the first place.

If this did happen it would effectively serve to justify the barriers that your nervous system had previously put in place, and you will subconsciously revert back to your comfort zone. You can see from this example why so many people fail to achieve their desired results regardless of how hard or how often they train.

To avoid this frustrating fate we're going to teach you exactly how to ease into your newfound flexibility and train your nervous system progressively to accept that it is not in any danger as a result of stretching its boundaries.

The third and final factor in the formula is to continually recreate the accepted envelope of movement that defines how much your muscles can stretch. All you need to do is…

REPEAT

The way to approach this is very much in line with the way you would learn any new skill: practice properly and often. Over time, as you continually hold a stretched out position for longer and longer periods, your nervous system will come to accept that as the new 'standard', and will no longer tense up when you reach that threshold. So, it follows that to make consistent progress you simply need to practice consistently.

These three underlying principles are made up of five highly effective techniques that have been scientifically proven to yield fast and permanent results.

We'll cover each of these methods in the coming chapters and gradually redraw the boundaries of your flexibility.

Stick with us; this is going to blow your mind.

"I use both dynamic and static stretching in my training. Flexibility is crucial to my fitness."

Samantha Stosur

4. STEP 1: ACHIEVING ZEN

We begin this tutorial with an important note on achieving Zen-like levels of relaxation! We previously mentioned the necessity to keep your mind relaxed in order to continually improve your flexibility. Let's expand on that concept.

Most of us have undoubtedly experienced the curious sensation of having muscles tighten after an intense emotional experience, such as being startled unexpectedly. This same concept applies where flexibility is concerned.

If you are not mentally 'in the zone' when you begin a stretching session, there is no way your muscles will play ball. We therefore need to set an example for our muscles to follow. Remember, you will always get out what you put in.

So what's the best method for reaching a Zen-like level of mind and muscle relaxation?

Unfortunately, there is no universal answer to this question that will solve everyone's flexibility issues, but there are most certainly several highly effective techniques we can pass along. Try them out, see what works and run with it. But before you do that, we must briefly touch on safety.

The very moment your mind, whether it is conscious or unconscious, detects even the slightest threat, your muscles will automatically tighten up as a defense mechanism. Naturally, there is very little you can do to reverse this action once it has occurred, but you can take measures to prevent it happening in the first place.

Take every possible precaution to make yourself as safe and as comfortable as possible before you dive into your routine. Remember, there is no physiological barrier between you and your desired range of movement; it's a mental game, and our perceived image of how unsafe or painful getting there might be is pivotal.

Therefore, go to whatever lengths you must to make yourself feel completely at ease when sliding into a stretch. Use a spotter, set some mats down, put on some calming music or whatever else works.

Generally speaking, if it puts your mind at ease, go ahead and do it. You'll be amazed just how quickly and completely your muscles will relax as soon as you remove any source of concern or worry from your external environment.

Another way to put your mind at ease while attempting new maneuvers stems from more traditional meditation and relaxation techniques that are now being employed across the sports and fitness industry.

You needn't go to the extremes of training with Tibetan monks, burning incense and chanting 'Om' in order to enjoy the benefits offered by the underpinning techniques that make up these ancient practices.

The primary components of these relaxation techniques involve being aware of and controlling your breathing, and interpreting your body's reactions through a technique known as biofeedback. We will explore these concepts of control in later sections. For now, just make sure you're nailing the basics and get yourself in the zone.

As for the intended targets and scope of this section, it's universal! Regardless of the method or technique that you employ to increase your flexibility, safety should always be a primary concern, because if you put yourself in danger your body will know about it, making the techniques and exercises null and void.

Trust us, it's perfectly acceptable to take extreme steps to ensure safety. If it eases your mind, and therefore muscular tension, then we wholeheartedly encourage you to do it. Furthermore, pushing your flexibility to its limits will naturally incur some degree of risk whatever you do. So, you can never be too careful.

Training your mind to exert more control over the tensioning and loosening of certain muscle groups takes time and practice, but this increased level of mental and physical control will work wonders for your flexibility regimen as you begin to push your limits.

Once you've got your external environment set up and your internal environment is rewarding you with calmness, you have already completed step one. Yup, believe it or not, you have already offered yourself the potential to stretch further and better simply by switching off the outside world and getting prepared.

Use this as a starting point for all of the techniques that follow. We'll start off simple, with a game of chicken.

"Slow it down, free the body. That's what it's about. Freedom of movement."

Conor McGregor

5. Step 2: A Game of Chicken

As covered in the previous chapter, the first step in our formula for leveling up your flexibility is to relax. We'll initially accomplish this through a technique that involves gradually increasing a stretch at a rate your nervous system is happy with.

In a nutshell, you will pick a stretch to hold and stay in that position until your muscles begin to relax. Once you begin to feel this, you will be able to gradually increase the stretch until you feel the tension return, and then start the process over.

Be sure to pick a position that you can hold for over a minute when starting off with this; as a beginner you will not fare well by picking something excruciatingly difficult and expecting your body to accept it right away.

Naturally, lower body stretches will be the prime target for many people. Think deep squats or seated groin stretches, for example. Remember, the key is to completely relax your body and mind to the point that you almost forget that you are stretching at all.

The Why

Remember that the muscle contractions you initially feel when stretching is simply the automatic protective response from your nervous system. If it detects your muscles moving outside their preset range of motion, it will let you know! If you continue to hold a stretch regardless of the alarm bells going off in your head, you will accomplish two pivotal goals:

First, you're allowing your nervous system to realize that the muscles are at the limit, or outside of their normal envelope, and yet no harm is being done. This is crucial in order for your body and mind to comprehend that abnormal muscle movement does not necessarily equate to injury.

The second victory is that of 'waiting out' your nervous system. Eventually, generally after just a few minutes, your muscles will no longer be able to maintain the amount of tension required to prevent further movement. At that moment, you will be able to slide a little deeper into the stretch until your body picks up on the new movement, and the process starts all over again.

Think of this as a game of chicken with your nervous system, one that you will always win so long as you have the patience to wait it out.

So, just as we are teaching your body that there is no damage associated with the new movement, we're also gently reassuring the nervous system that its automatic response to tighten muscles is no longer required as the muscles elongate. This means the more progress you make, the less your nervous system will try to intervene in future, allowing your results to snowball all the way to superhuman!

Please remember, patience is the key factor in this exercise. If you are rushed, or try to force the tempo of your muscle relaxation, your body will fight you tooth and nail for as long as possible. So don't forget the first key: relax.

Don't stare at a clock or count down in your head. Try thinking about your day, or what tomorrow's plans are; anything to take your mind away from the peculiar positioning of your muscles. Thinking of food is also a surefire method to distract your brain, just don't get up for a snack!

This will naturally take practice, but as soon as you reach the stage where your focus is shifted away from the tension in your muscles, you'll be surprised at just how quickly they will loosen up and allow you to slide deeper into the stretch.

To conclude this 'waiting out' of muscular tension method, we'd like to remind you of its intended targets and scope. As we briefly mentioned earlier, lower body muscles are the prime targets for this technique, specifically the hips and legs.

You might find that trying to hold an upper body stretch for long periods of time is too difficult, therefore we recommend utilizing this technique primarily to open up your lower body mobility to greater levels, which will naturally promote increased strength and performance thanks to your new and improved range of motion.

Lastly, we strongly advise against using this technique on your back. You have probably experienced the stiffness and cramps that come as a result of holding your back in a certain position for long period of time, perhaps even from a poor sitting or sleeping posture. Waiting out the tension on your back is a sure fire way to invite those aches and pains, or possibly worse.

This is due to the key role that supportive ligaments play in keeping your spine in proper alignment, and prolonged stretching can throw that supportive system out of sync. So again, focus on the lower body here, and try some upper body if you find it comfortable and effective. After all, everybody is different.

So, we've covered the what and the why behind this technique, so let's get to the how!

THE HOW

A few stretches to try out with this method include deep squats, seated groin stretches, pigeon pose, runners stretch, and of course, the splits! For reference, these will all play a part in opening up your hip flexors, and increased mobility in this area will lead to phenomenal performance increases throughout your entire lower body and core.

WAITING OUT TENSION STEPS

1. Select a familiar stretch that you can maintain for a good few minutes. You'll find some examples in chapter 12, but be sure to warm up first.

2. Sink into the stretch until you feel the target muscles tighten at your regular limit of movement. You will soon realize that this is not actually your limit at all!

3. Stay in this position and allow yourself to relax. Daydream, breathe calmly, close your eyes or whatever helps. Forget about the time, you're not up against the clock here.

4. As your muscles get tired of fighting back, normally within a few minutes, they will begin to relax. Take this opportunity to gradually increase the stretch.

5. When the muscle tension returns at the new boundary of movement, repeat steps 3 and 4. When you feel you have reached your absolute limit, you can bring it back to the start and perform another set.

Tip: Gently jiggle, roll or massage your way into more comfortable positions from time to time in order to aid relaxation.

6. Step 3: Flexing for Flexibility

The next method to give your flexibility a nudge in the right direction involves flexing your muscles during a stretch. This may sound counterproductive, but it works wonders for breaking barriers. If you want the full, fancy name, then take a deep breath because it's a mouthful:

Proprioceptive Neuromuscular Facilitation (we'll just stick with PNF) is a remarkably effective way to make consistent gains as you attempt to increase your overall flexibility and range of motion. What's more, this method also develops and strengthens your muscles at the same time, so what's not to like?

PNF in a Nutshell

As you know, when you stretch your muscles will automatically tighten in response. This is your overprotective nervous system taking charge with the best intentions to guard you from what it perceives as imminent injury. Here's a hack to override the reflex

Once you reach the limit that the muscle will allow, you'll now fire it up and briefly but forcefully contract it. After a second or two, you will release the contraction and find that the muscle relaxes back into a stretch that is deeper than the one you started with. Nope, it's not witchcraft, just simple science again.

In essence, we're pulling the wool over your nervous system's eyes with a sleight of hand trick. As you begin the stretching process, the automatic muscle tensioning reflex will kick in, and you will soon reach the point where your nervous system is under the impression that it is straining or contracting the muscles to their limit and lock down will commence. However, you can temporarily throw your nervous system out of sync by contracting that muscle even further yourself.

This causes your nervous system to briefly go 'offline', because it thinks you are doing its job for it, and it takes time for this reflex to reset. Therefore, as soon as you release the contraction and sink even deeper into the stretch, while your hoodwinked nervous system is still recovering from being disengaged, the muscle will relax significantly, thus allowing you the opportunity to extend the stretch further. Voilà, you just duped your nervous system into increasing your flexibility!

Of course, it will wise up pretty quickly and re-engage the reflex to tighten the muscle. At this point you'll be slightly deeper into the stretch and can repeat the same process to increase it further and allow your body to get used to its new range of movement. So, why do we need this technique at all when we've already got a perfectly good one?

THE WHY

Recall our formula for success earlier in this guide. This technique works towards the principle of 'training' your body to realize that there are new limits to the amount that your muscles can stretch, and that injury is not imminent when gently pushing those limits. This is a step beyond simply overcoming the threshold in the first place.

PNF, or isometric stretching, will also be a potent tool for developing your muscular strength and flexibility together. Thus far, the stretching and flexibility methods we've presented have involved simply relaxing the muscle in order to stretch it a little farther, however, relaxing a muscle does not build strength, and your nervous system demands that strength and flexibility be developed in tandem.

Consider, for example, an individual rendered unconscious by injury or anesthesia. When the conscious mind is no longer controlling muscle movement, the unconscious person's limbs can be manually rotated through extreme angles without even a hint of difficulty, because the nervous system is 'offline' and unable to determine whether or not the muscles can cope with this movement.

However, as soon as this person wakes up and the conscious mind retakes the reins this boundless flexibility is once again constrained to its predefined envelope, because the nervous system knows that the muscles are not strong enough to cope with the new range of movement.

Here your nervous system is essentially regulating your flexibility based on the strength of the muscles in question. If your system does not believe that you have the strength to control increased flexibility, then it will not allow further progress.

For a real world example, visualize a set of muscles, in the shoulder for example, that have excellent mobility but low overall strength. You're rock climbing, and you feel that you could contort that shoulder in an extreme position to reach a certain hold, but as soon as you try to support yourself while in that extreme position, the muscles give out and the shoulder buckles. Hopefully you aren't too high up!

With this example it's easy to visualize how the connective tissue or the joint itself could be seriously damaged if you did not possess the strength to hold your shoulder in that position, even if you could achieve it momentarily.

It is imperative, then, to use this technique not just to achieve greater ROM, but also to strengthen the muscles while they are in these new positions to ensure that you can remain in control for every single degree of freedom that you achieve. This is effectively training the nervous system to accept that you are capable of operating within this new range of motion, allowing you to increase strength and flexibility without interruption.

THE HOW

This is where isometric stretching comes in. Isometrics, traditionally, is the practice of using immovable objects for resistance in order to increase strength. For the purposes of building strength and flexibility, we simply need to stretch to our boundaries, and then contract the muscle to achieve the same effect.

Consider the common 'plank' exercise for example; this movement is very taxing and can build remarkable core strength even though no actual movement takes place. This is because you are essentially pitting your muscles against a static opponent, one that provides infinite resistance, which is the very same concept we are applying here.

The more you practice this stretching technique the more your muscles will develop at the same time. So, next time your nervous system tries to determine if you're strong enough to handle increased flexibility, you can say 'step back, I got this!'

As for the target muscle groups and scope for this method, you'll find that it can be more widely applied than the waiting out of tension technique. Here, we can flex our muscles to achieve increased flexibility with nearly any primary muscle group.

PROPRIOCEPTIVE NEUROMUSCULAR FACILITATION (PNF) STEPS:

1. Begin the stretch for your target muscle group.

2. Stretch to the point where your muscles automatically tighten.

3. At this point, fire those muscles up and contract them gradually but forcibly.

4. Hold the fully contracted muscles for 1 to 2 seconds then release.

5. Your nervous system is now offline, you can gently sink deeper into the stretch.

6. Repeat as required and feel like a boss!

Tip: For greatest effect, remember to relax before you begin. See a physician regarding stretches on your back to ensure you are operating safely!

7. STEP 4: BREATHE, BELIEVE, ACHIEVE

So far we've covered general relaxation along with using tension to ease deeper into a stretch. It's time to toss regulated breathing into the mix, something that will drastically improve your results.

Picture yourself during a particularly intense workout; perhaps a combination of strength and cardio with little rest between the two. Your heart is pounding, your target muscles are brimming with lactic acid and burning up, the exercise is becoming more and more difficult to perform with every rep.

You begin to breathe heavier and faster, feel sweat racing down your brow and then, finally, you smash out that final rep and, thank the good lord, it's all over! Now you're standing there, gasping for air, and your heart feels close to popping a rib or two out of place. What's the first thing you do?

If you're an athlete you've probably been taught since little league to place your hands on your head, open up those lungs and regain control of your breathing. If you're not an athlete you probably do it a little less gracefully, likely curled up in the fetal position gasping like a fish out of water, but the end goal is the same. Let's take a look at why.

THE WHY

OK, for the smartasses out there, we breathe to remain alive. But to truly understand how this relates to our ability to become more flexible, we need to look a little deeper.

By taking steady, controlled, breaths the rest of your body will fall in line and effectively 'calm down'. Your heart rate will decrease, your muscles will relax, and your body will begin to return to business as usual.

This is an excellent example of the remarkable control that breathing exerts over the rest of our automatic processes. This is possible due to the fact that breathing is the only bodily process that bridges the gap between automatic and voluntary functions.

By now it's been well established that the vast majority of bodily functions that regulate your flexibility are maddeningly involuntary, automatic processes that our old friend the nervous system controls in the background.

Technically, breathing falls under this category too. Imagine how strange it would be if you had to consciously remember to take in oxygen and expel carbon dioxide every few seconds. We'd scarcely have time to get anything else done! Thankfully this process is largely placed on autopilot, but it can still be hijacked by the conscious mind and utilized for our benefit. In plain English, this means we can change our breathing and change our state completely at will.

This, in turn, gives you the power to control your muscular tension, heart rate, and a myriad of other functions as they all take their marching orders from your breathing.

This type of control is known in technical terms as 'biofeedback'. Essentially, you are training yourself to become aware of your breathing, detect the effects it is having on your body, and re-adjust accordingly to achieve the desired results.

Several advanced meditation techniques around the world are founded on this method, because controlling your breathing is key to controlling your overall state.

For our purposes, this can be used as follows:

THE HOW

First you'll begin to stretch as you normally would and sink down to the point where your muscle tension prevents further movement. Then you'll tense up your entire body from toe to jaw, not just the target muscles, take a deep breath and hold it in.

The smart cookies among you will have realized that we are combining PNF with these breathing techniques to create a sort of super formula for relaxation now. For the rest of you, do try to keep up!

An excellent analogy is to imagine your body as a beach ball and that you are drawing in breath to inflate it. Now hold that tension, and your breath, for a second or two, and then pop! Let it all out at once and imagine the balloon deflating.

Relax all your muscles at the same time, and exhale deeply and completely. Everything relaxes instantly; the beach ball in your mind goes limp and flexible, as does your body! You will sink a little deeper into your stretch as your entire body relaxes. Aim to add a little more with each cycle, and repeat until you reach a plateau.

A word of caution on breathing: the deep breaths used here have the potential to cause hyperventilation. If you begin to feel lightheaded, breathe normally for a few seconds between sets and take a break between each cycle. Of course, if you are asthmatic or have any kind of respiratory condition, see a doctor to discuss what is safe for you to try.

The controlled breathing technique can be applied to any muscle group that you are inclined to relax with the PNF method. As you will have noticed, the main differences between the two are the inclusion of the breathing technique, and the fact that you are tensing your entire body instead of just the muscles that you are trying to stretch.

This is a crucial step in the process, so don't dismiss it! Tensing your entire body sets the stage for everything, both your body and mind, to relax in one fell swoop when you release the breath. This relaxation process is a good deal more far-reaching than the targeted muscle tension in PNF, and will therefore most likely yield improved results.

CONTROLLED BREATHING STEPS:

1. Begin the stretch for your target muscle group.

2. Stretch to the point where your muscles automatically tighten.

3. At this point, take a deep breath. Recall the beach ball analogy.

4. Tense your entire body forcibly at the same time.

5. Hold the tension and breath for a couple of seconds then release and exhale deeply.

6. Sink deeper into the stretch and repeat as required.

Super important: If you are using this technique on your back, do not hold the relaxed position for more than a second or two as this will put strain on the ligaments instead of the muscles. You don't want to be hunched over like a shrimp for too long while your back muscles are offline.

To come back up from this kind of position, it's also a good idea to move slowly into a squat position and then push up from there, rather than putting all the strain on your back. We cannot stress enough the importance of good spine health. Look after your back and it will look after you!

This technique should be fairly simple to master, so give it a try and see if it works for you. We all respond differently to different stimuli, so if you're not feeling this, check out the next technique and compare results.

8. Step 5: Overload and Override

We're certain you will find waiting out tension, PNF and controlled breathing to be excellent tools for your flexibility and strength training. However, if these methods of relaxation and control don't take you far enough over a longer period of time, you can always up the ante with the 'overload and override' (O&O) technique.

As you may have deduced from the name, this technique involves manually overriding your nervous system's response by overloading your muscles to the point of exhaustion.

To accomplish this, you will begin to stretch, and push yourself until you hit the point of muscle tension that prevents any further movement. At this point, you will ease into tensing the muscles in question, keeping your effort to about 60% of your max strength.

You will hold the tension for as long as you physically can while taking steady, shallow breaths and gradually increasing your exertion level on the tensed muscles. When your mental gauge clicks into 'for the love of God, let it stop!' mode, releasing the tension entirely will allow a feeling of relaxation wash over you, so you can slide deeper into your stretch as the muscles give out.

The Why

This goes a step further than the standard PNF technique, which simply hoodwinks your nervous system into letting you increase a stretch. O&O actually physically exhausts your muscles to the point where they simply cannot offer any further resistance to your stretching after you've release the tension.

As always, your nervous system automatically takes charge when you start to approach the border of your flexibility limit, and will tense the offending muscle to prevent further movement at first. However, this form of restrictive tension takes energy and strength to maintain. Therefore, when you one-up your nervous system by actively tensing those muscles to an even greater degree you quickly drain your energy reserves. Depending on your own physiology and the muscles you are training, the timescale varies and you will need to experiment to discover your own tolerances.

As soon as you hit the point where you cannot physically hold the tension any longer and begin to slide deeper into the stretch, your nervous system is also out of energy and there's nothing it can do to stop you! You will find that this is a higher intensity version of stretching than what we've covered so far, but that just makes it more effective.

As with the PNF method, O&O comes with the added benefit of building muscle strength and stamina over the course of your routine, but to a greater degree. Previously with the PNF or controlled breathing methods, we only taxed the muscles for a couple of seconds before releasing the tension, here we're taking them all the way.

THE HOW

In this case, we're holding the tension for as long as physically possible. Remember the planking example? It's a very similar concept, except now we are planking until we crash to the ground. This significantly increases the amount of muscular development, with the end result of huge gains in flexibility and strength. Perfect for mastering calisthenics!

It will take practice and repetition to determine exactly what amount of tension and time is required for each muscle group. This varies from person to person, so keep track of your progress to find the sweet spot for forced relaxation stretching.

This can be used for any of the same muscle groups as controlled breathing or PNF methods. Hips and shoulders are the prime targets, but forearms, biceps, calves, and generally any other stiff muscle can benefit from this movement too.

Another word of warning concerning your back, however:

We cannot recommend this technique for use on the back muscles because it will again place strain on areas you really want to protect.

OVERLOAD AND OVERRIDE STEPS

1. Begin the stretch for your target muscle group.

2. Stretch to the point where your muscles automatically tighten.

3. At this point, begin to take steady and shallow breaths.

4. Tension the muscle to about 30-60% of your maximum effort.

5. Hold the tension for as long as physically possible, as if you were resisting someone pushing the other way, and release when the muscle physically gives way.

6. Sink deeper into the stretch in a controlled manner and repeat as required.

Remember: This technique is a marathon, not a sprint. It takes as long as it takes!

"Practice puts brains in your muscles."

Sam Snead

9. THE SECRET WEAPON

We have one final weapon in the arsenal, reserved only for the most extreme cases. This last line of attack is known as the 'clasp-knife' technique, on account of the way that the sudden shift of a muscle or limb resembles the snap closure of a clasp-knife after sufficient pressure is applied. Oh yes, this is serious sausages right here.

Warning: This is an **extreme** method of stretching that should be kept behind closed doors unless absolutely required. Most people should have no need of such drastic measures. If you have a strict goal to meet and need that extra inch, then do everything else again and do it properly! This final method will get you there, but it is a last resort, not a shortcut for the impatient.

The process we'll use here is almost identical to the forced relaxation method, with one small modification. Instead of tensing your muscles to 60% of your maximum effort, we're going all the way to 100%, and adding weight.

This is the secret weapon of many a coach and trainer, one which enables gymnasts and other professionals to contort themselves into human-pretzel hybrid form without so much as flinching. This technique requires a special expertise to pull off. For this reason, clasp-knife stretching should only ever be performed under the supervision of a coach or trainer who has experience with it.

THE WHY

By hitting maximum capacity we're attempting to utilize another automatic reflex that your nervous system has in stock. Up to this point the only reflex we've experienced is the automatic muscle tensioning that occurs when your push muscles to their flexibility limits. However, another reflex exists that actually causes your muscles to go totally limp! It is this reflex that we will engage with the clasp-knife method.

As we know by now, whenever a muscle is put under a great deal of strain the nervous system will automatically tense the muscle to prevent further movement. However, if the strain on the muscle continues to increase, eventually the nervous system will reach a point where it would rather completely relax the muscle than risk damage occurring to the critical supporting structure, effectively 'taking one for the team', if you will. As a result of this process, the target muscle becomes yours to command and you are able to massively increase the level of stretching and flexibility.

Now, don't worry, we're not actually going to injure you here. Like any good program, your body has an ample margin of safety coded in. Tissue and tendons are stronger than muscle so, by the time the muscle gives out, you can rest assured that you are still some way off putting those other areas in danger.

That being said, you can expect a good deal of pain when using this technique. After all, we are pushing to the point where your nervous system detects the extreme pain and strain in your muscles and believes that there is no choice but to relax the muscle.

THE HOW

Remember, this is a last resort when all other options fail to get you to your flexibility goals. This particular technique can be used on the same muscle groups as the forced relaxation method. However, this very much depends on your personal pain tolerance and the sensitivity of your muscles.

Perhaps this technique could be the final push you need to achieve a deep squat, but is unbearable for your groin stretches. Take it easy to start with and determine your own tolerances for each muscle. Of course, don't even think about using it on your back.

Most people will never need to unleash this weapon and those who do are normally either too impatient to stick with the previous methods, or competitive athletes dealing with extremely fine margins. Determine which one you are and ask yourself if you really need to take these measures before you proceed to the below steps.

CLASP-KNIFE STEPS

1. Stretch the target muscle and bring it to the point of automatic tightening.

2. At this point, begin to take steady and shallow breaths.

3. Take a few seconds to gradually tense the muscle from 60% up to 100%. Where the last stretch was a marathon, this is more of a sprint from hereon.

4. Your coach will add weight now. Hold full tension until you experience muscle spasms. It should give out within around 10-20 seconds. If not, reset manually and try again.

5. Once the muscle gives out, release all the tension at once in a controlled manner, exhaling deeply as you have learned previously. Remember, you are a beach ball!

6. Sink deeper into the stretch for around 5 seconds and repeat as required.

A Word on Weights

The clasp-knife can be thought of as 'juiced up' overload and override. By adding weight to the equation and ramping your contractions up to 100% effort, you should be able to achieve your goal.

This will need to be done under the direction, and quite literally under the weight of a coach or trainer. They will apply force to the tensed muscle and this increased load will effectively be the straw that breaks the camel's back.

It is possible to perform weighted stretches yourself, but you may find it more difficult. For example, you could perform deep squats with a Bulgarian bag on your shoulders. The problem here arises after the stretch has taken place.

It is much safer and more effective to have a professional coach provide the weight so that they can intuitively release it when you finish a the stretch. You may find it difficult to get out of certain situations if you are handling the weights yourself.

If you do go down this route, please think forward and ensure you're not weighting yourself into a position you can't get out of! At the very least, have a spotter on hand.

Despite the grizzly nature of this technique it is, in fact, safe to perform when done properly. However, please do remember that this is a final measure for experienced athletes who have already completed all the previous steps and need that extra 1%.

10. Stretch Smart

We always recommend working one on one with a certified and reputable professional, at least for your first few sessions, because they will be able to assess your individual case and ensure you start off on the right foot.

It's absolutely maddening to see some of the bad habits people persist with simply because they were never taught otherwise. While we can't provide individual advice, there are some very important pointers we can provide.

Stretch the Right Spots

Notice how we've only discussed muscles throughout this entire guide? There's a good reason for that. Tendons and other connective tissues are not designed to be stretched or exerted beyond their normal stability duties. They are meant to function as support girders of sorts for all your joints. They keep everything aligned and rotating the way they should.

Consequently, connective tissue has very little play or flexibility, because how often do you pull apart your knee joints for kicks and giggles? It just doesn't happen! So, your connective tissue and ligaments are NOT designed to stretch. If they do, even just a fractional amount, a whole host of problems may develop.

Such issues include elongation, scar tissue from micro-tears, and weakening. In essence, the ligament would no longer offer the rigid support that it used to, which leaves the door wide open for the joint to be compromised and injured. Long story short, you need to avoid straining your ligaments.

This brings us to a slightly gray area in the world of stretching. Just how can you be sure that you're stretching the muscles and not the ligaments in that same area?

The first step is to be aware of where your connective tissue is located around the joints, and the second step is to recognize the difference between the 'pull' of muscle stretching and the outright pain of connective tissue strain.

For example, if you're in the middle of a hamstring stretch and pain begins to build up directly behind or on the side of your knee, you'll know that you strayed into tendon territory, so ease back.

Generally speaking, if you begin to feel the sharp pain of connective tissue strain, try to bend the corresponding joint slightly, in the above case the knee. This should ease the pressure on your connective tissue and redirect the force of the stretch into your muscles, i.e. the hamstring in this example.

Furthermore, always take care to complete a stretch in the correct manner. Double check your posture and motion in order to put the least amount of stain as possible on your connective ligaments, and make sure you've studied a body map of the areas you're working on so you can recognize and distinguish between muscle and ligament.

DEALING WITH INJURIES

For athletes, or anyone else highly invested in their fitness, injuries can be one of the most irritating and depressing issues to develop. Mentally, you're all set and ready to go: you have the energy, the time, and the motivation, but your body isn't working properly. Remarkably frustrating, but we still have to keep those muscles moving!

When a muscle gets injured, it automatically contracts to protect itself from further damage. This is useful for keeping swelling down, and informing you that a problem exists. However, muscle contractions also limit blood flow to that area, and nourishing blood is exactly what the muscle needs to heal. What's more, constant contraction also hits the reset button on that muscle's flexibility envelope. With little use during the injured period, the muscle slowly begins to degrade, build scar tissue and lose its strength. Consequently, your nervous system will restrict its flexibility even more, as covered in previous sections. This is a cycle you want to nip in the bud.

So, in order to increase blood flow to the muscle, promote healing, retain strength and maintain flexibility we have to stretch the injured muscle. Yes, it hurts, but it has to be done. Of course, the first step to treating an injury is generally the interventional 'R.I.C.E' (Rest, Ice, Compression, Elevation) method applied immediately after the injury is sustained, but it's good to begin stretching soon after, even within 48 hours.

Disclaimer: Hopefully you never get injured, but if you do, be smart about it and see a professional physician before doing anything else. As valuable as the advice in this book is, it is no substitute for standing in front of a human being who can assess your own individual case and advise on a bespoke course of treatment. Use this guide only as a supplement to professional advice, not a substitute for it.

For injured muscles, it's recommended that you use less intensive stretching methods, such as contrast breathing and PNF techniques. In this case the muscles are extremely sensitive, so very gradually ease into the stretches. That means you should slowly slide into the stretch, and tense your muscles one step at a time to ease the shock to your system. This slow but steady pace of stretching will help to keep the muscle moving and increase blood flow, but limit the sudden and intense strain that accompanies the clasp knife and other harsh methods.

Overall, just be smart with injuries. Listen to your body and don't push it too far, but keep it active enough to prevent muscle degradation.

STRETCHING FOR LIFE

Naturally, we are at our most limber as children. However, we adults have something the kids don't: mental discipline and the patience to complete the more intensive and time consuming stretches that we've covered in this guide, such as contrast breathing and PNF.

Therefore, children are generally encouraged to complete more active stretching that can be completed on the go, while playing, and which requires little time or thought.

A word of warning, however: children's' backs and shoulders (under the age of about 12) are notoriously sensitive. So we cannot recommend straining those at all. On the flip side, their lower bodies are remarkably flexible and childhood is the best time to develop excellent hip mobility, something that can plague us all later in life.

Of course, as we knock on, inevitable aches and pains creep into the picture. This is the prime time to utilize all of the tools presented in this guide. Waiting out the tension, PNF, contrast breathing, and forced relaxation will push you past your wildest flexibility fantasies.

Lastly, women that are pregnant should not jump right into the stretching routines we've described. It's always recommended to consult with your doctor first as your body chemistry changes throughout pregnancy.

More specifically, the amount of relaxin released into your system affects many of your joints and can throw your overall reflexes and range of motion slightly out of whack. It's best to consult a professional who can assess your own case.

So, are you ready to put your newfound knowledge to the test? Let's get started with a quick warm-up. Yes, that's right, we warm up for stretching too!

11. WARM-UP & PREPARATION

Whether you are a seasoned stretcher or a complete newbie it is essential to prepare properly if you want to achieve stunning results. Let's go through some gentle exercises designed to prime your muscles for stretching while increasing range of motion.

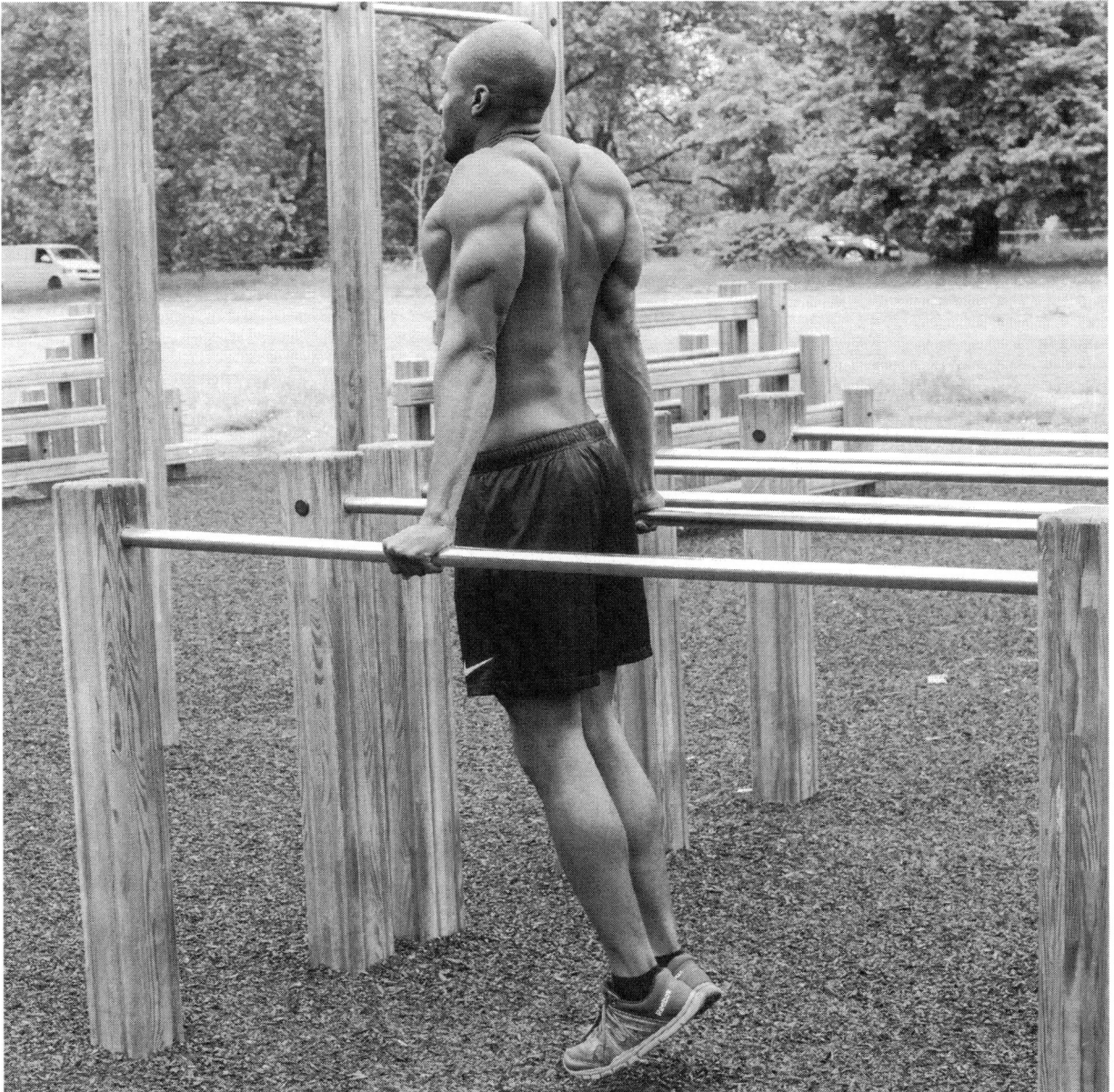

3 REASONS TO WARM UP

1. Your muscles will pool with blood, aiding relaxation and allowing you to maximize the potential of every stretch.

2. The risk of getting injured during training is minimized, meaning you won't have to cut sessions short or drop out entirely due to niggles or tears.

3. Range of motion increases enabling you to push your body to new limits. As you scale up in this way you will gain unprecedented strength and capability.

Some people consider warming up to be a waste of time, but if you're not willing to put in that little extra effort per session then we would have to question your commitment to mastering your fitness in the first place.

When you stop thinking of a warm-up as a chore and see the serious value it brings, it will revolutionize your workout and help you along the way to results you never thought were possible.

TIMING

If you are stretching post-workout, which you should be, then you are likely to be fairly well warmed up in some areas already. However, your stretching program may include muscles which aren't always included in your regular workouts, so it's good practice to give them a little wake-up call before you begin.

If some days of your stretching schedule fall on rest days when you are not working out, you must make double sure that your muscles are warm, nourished and ready to roll.

The whole process need not take more than a few minutes, and consists of three simple stages. First up we'll start with some basic mobility and motion.

MOBILITY

The first thing you need to do before stretching is loosen up the target areas you will be hitting. This doesn't need to be too strenuous, and there are no hard and fast rules. Generally speaking, just try to isolate the area with easy, controlled movements.

You will find some example exercises designed to warm up some of the key muscle groups and increase range of motion in the following pages. Cherry pick the exercises that are suitable and add your own in where needed.

Remember: This book is designed to create flexibility through stretching. While we can cover some essential mobility exercises, we don't have the scope to include them all. Use the mobility exercises in the coming pages as a guideline and build your own warm-up routine over time. Don't rush it, and don't skip it.

ISOMETRICS

The second step in preparing a muscle to be stretched is a short isometric contraction. This will cause the muscle to act like a sponge, drawing in a fresh batch of nourishing blood to prime the area for stretching.

For example, if you are stretching your glutes, squeeze them together hard as if you are trying to crack an egg between them! Hold for 30-60 seconds and then shake it out.

BREATHING

Remember that relaxation is key to a good stretch, so always allow your heart rate to return to normal and regain a steady rate of breathing before you begin.

You don't need to spend any significant amount of time here, just take a few breaths and compose yourself before you go into a stretch.

Upper Body

Your body may not quite be accustomed to the rigors of stretching combined with calisthenics, so spend 5-10 minutes going through the following, paying special attention to the areas of the body you plan to work on during your stretching session.

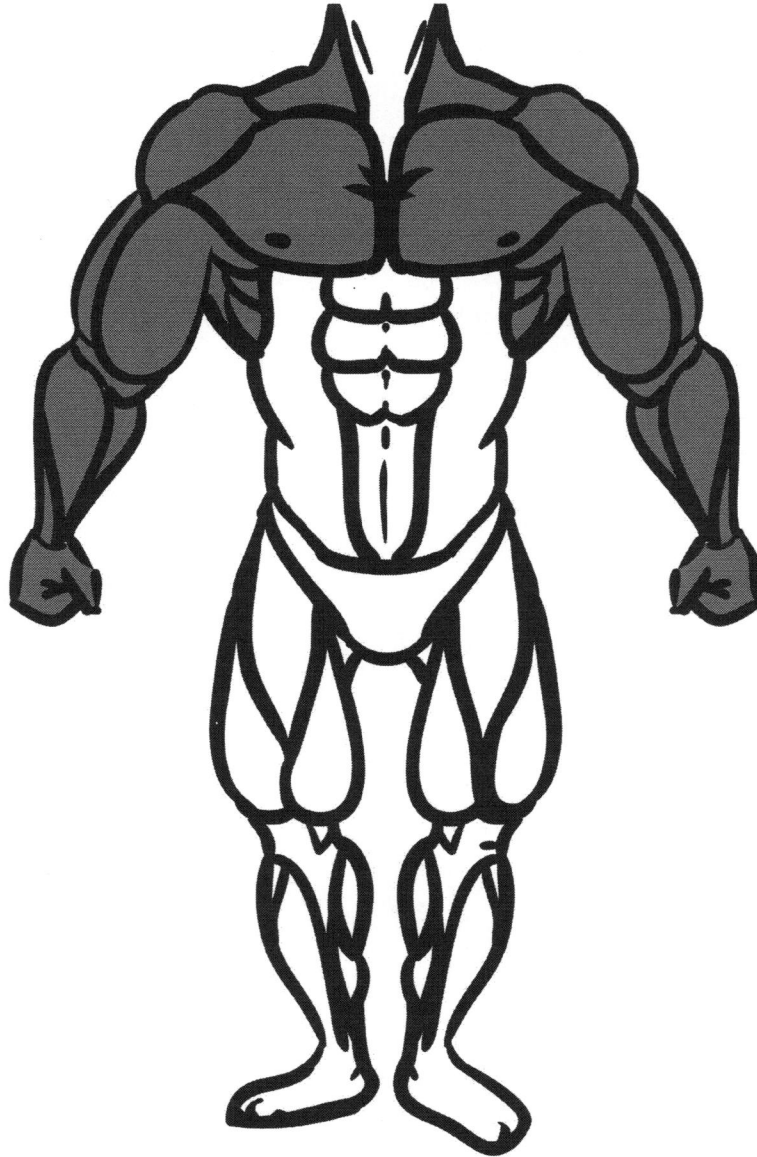

WRIST ROTATES

Your wrists are taxed in almost every calisthenics exercise, so try this simple warm-up to keep them strong and safe.

Perform: 10 seconds in each direction.

1. Extend your arms straight out in front of you.

2. Rotate your wrists clockwise for 10 seconds.

3. Switch directions and go again.

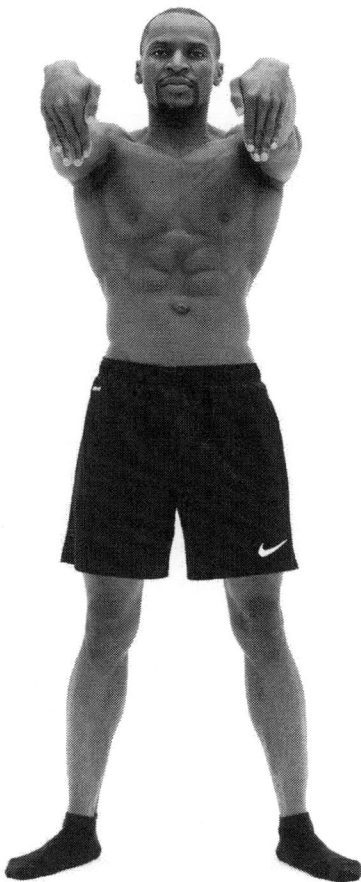 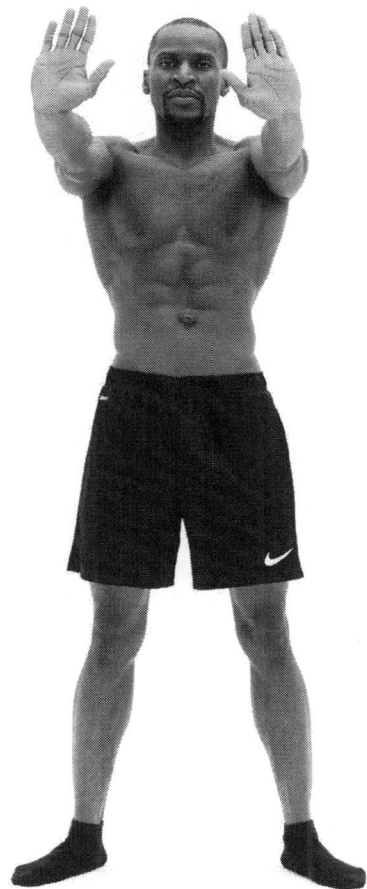

SHOULDER ROTATES

This is a simple but effective warm-up for the rotator cuff and shoulders.

Perform: 10 seconds in each direction.

1. Stand firm and extend both arms straight out to your sides.

2. Rotate arms forwards for 10 seconds.

3. Stop and do the same in reverse.

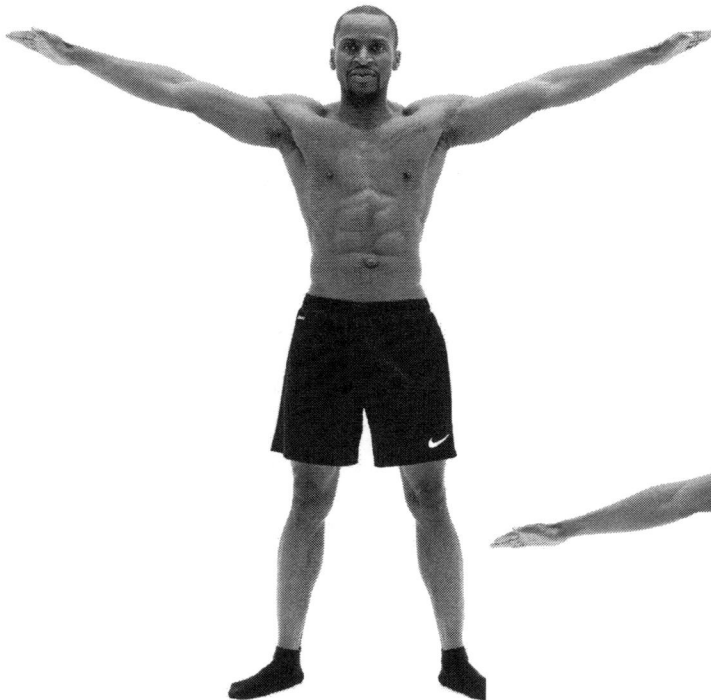
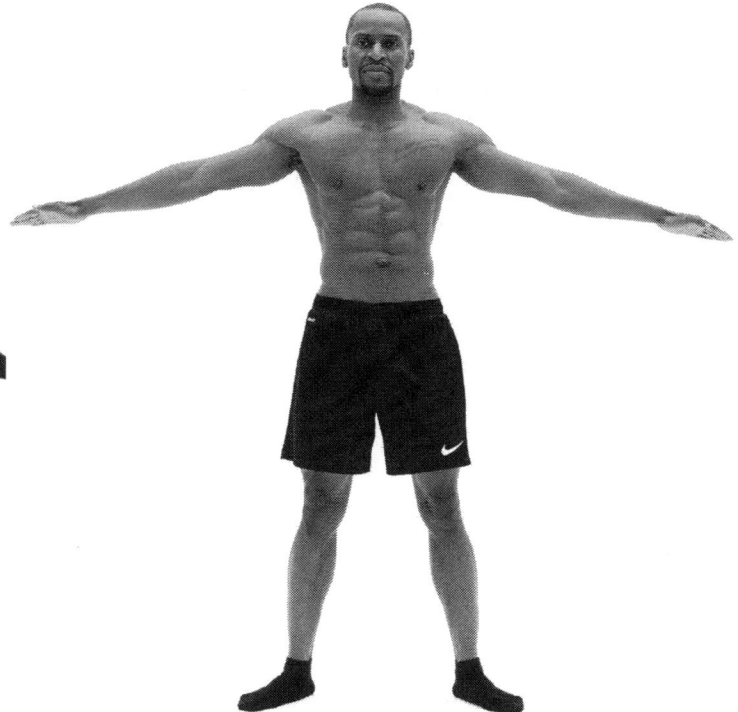

SHOULDER DISLOCATES

Don't panic, the clue isn't actually in the name this time! Your shoulders won't really pop out during this exercise, but they may still be a little uncomfortable at first. Since you will be opening up your shoulders, back, chest and arms here you will probably feel tightness in one or more areas.

Perform: 2 sets of 8 repetitions.

You will need: a long, lightweight bar.

1. Stand up straight, feet shoulder width apart, hands a little wider apart on the bar with an overhand grip (palms down).

2. Lift the bar up directly over your head and in one smooth motion bring it down to rest on your lower back, keeping your elbows locked at all times.

3. Reverse the movement, bringing the bar back to the front of your body to complete one rep.

You may struggle with this at first, so try sliding your hands wider apart along the bar until you find a position that allows you to perform the movement without bending your arms.

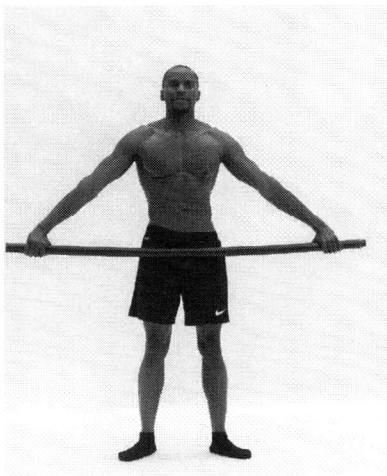

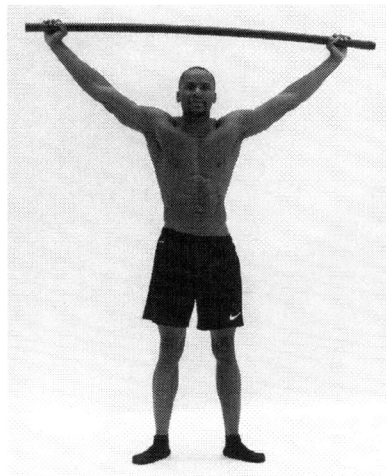

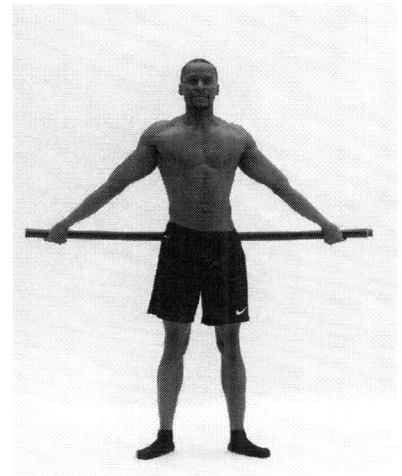

SCAPULA PUSH-UP

The scapula push-up is an excellent way to prepare your upper body for a beating. In particular, this will mobilize the muscles in your upper back and shoulders.

Perform: 8-10 repetitions.

1. Get into push-up position (see push-ups if unsure), placing your knees on the floor if you are just starting out.

2. Keeping your elbows locked and arms straight, let your chest sink towards the floor and squeeze your scapulae together at the same time.

3. With your elbows still locked, reverse this movement, lifting your chest back up and separating your scapula so that your back arches and your spine rises.

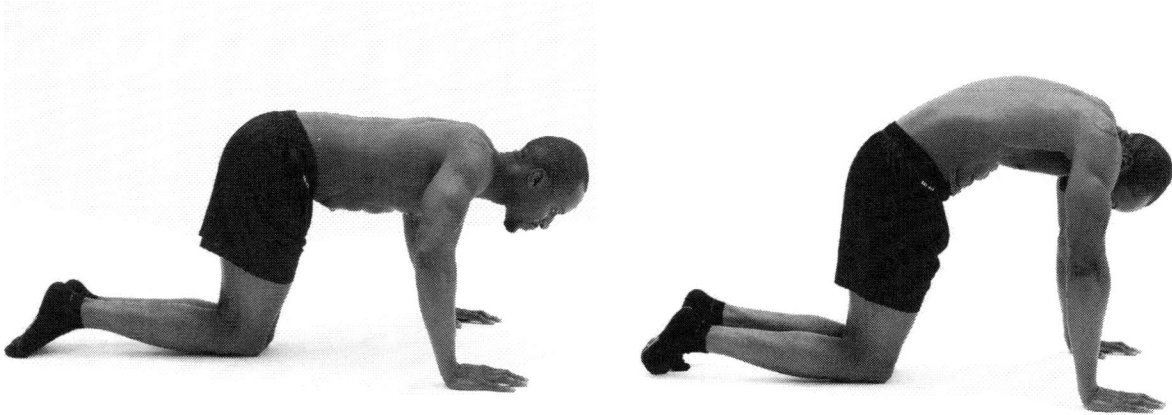

SCAPULA PULL-UP

The clue is in the name again; we'll be working your scapula and upper back here to great effect with an outstanding strengthening mobility exercise.

Perform: 8-10 repetitions.

You will need: a pull-up bar.

1. Grasp the bar overhand and allow yourself to hang with your arms and body totally straight, feet off the floor.

2. Relax, aiming to get your shoulders to touch your ears so your scapulae are elevated.

3. Keeping your arms and elbows locked in position; try to pull your scapulae downward.

4. Hold for 1-2 seconds and then lower back down to the starting position.

The movement involved in this exercise is so subtle that it is best demonstrated with good old-fashioned arrows! You may find this movement very difficult initially, but as with all things your mobility and control will improve over time so stick at it.

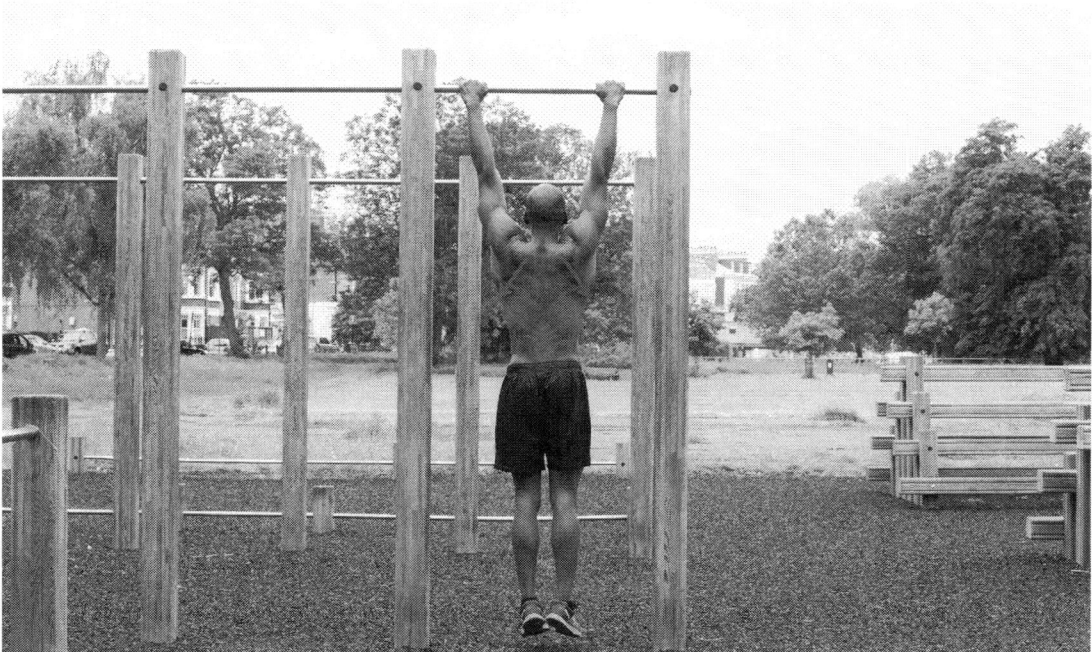

SCAPULA DIP

This motion will fire up your shoulders and give you greater range of movement for 'pushing' exercises such as, well, push-ups!

Perform: 8-10 repetitions.

You will need: parallel bars or dip station.

1. Grab the bars and lock your elbows, lifting your feet up and supporting your body-weight in a neutral position.

2. Keeping your elbows locked and arms straight, sink your body down aiming to get your shoulders to meet your ears (or as close as you can).

3. With your arms still locked straight, push back upwards as high as possible, effectively trying to get your shoulders and ears as far apart as you are able.

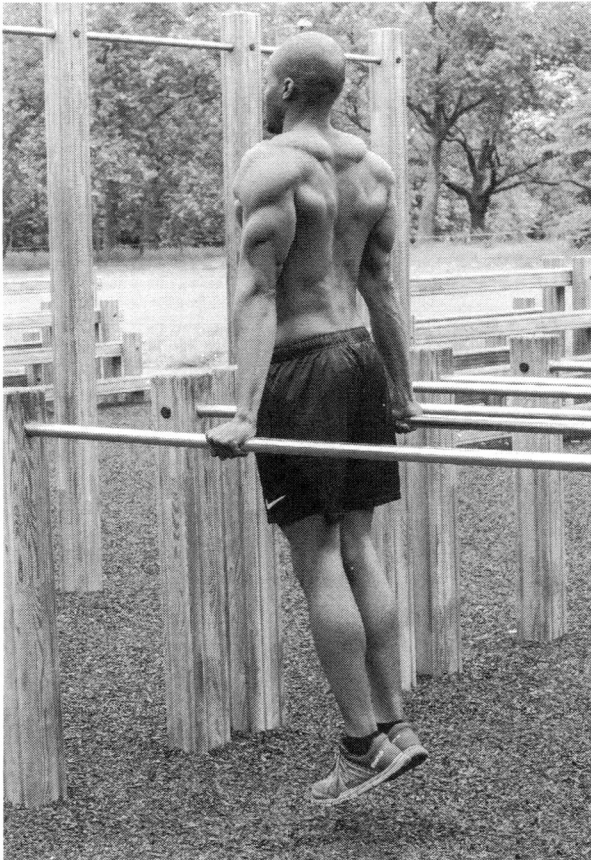

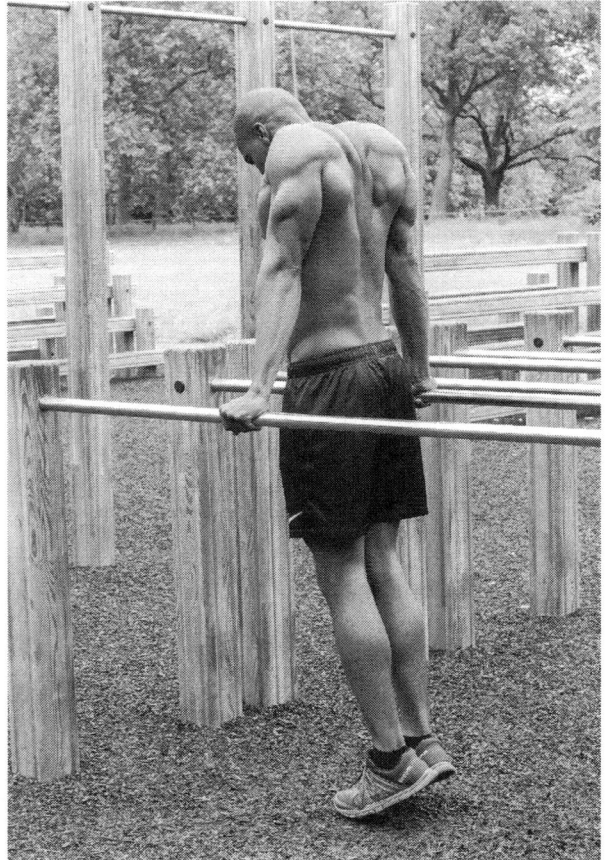

CORE

The core not only helps support the spine, but also plays a starring role in both exercise and everyday life. You will be glad to know that warming up the core is nice and quick to address, so let's get to it.

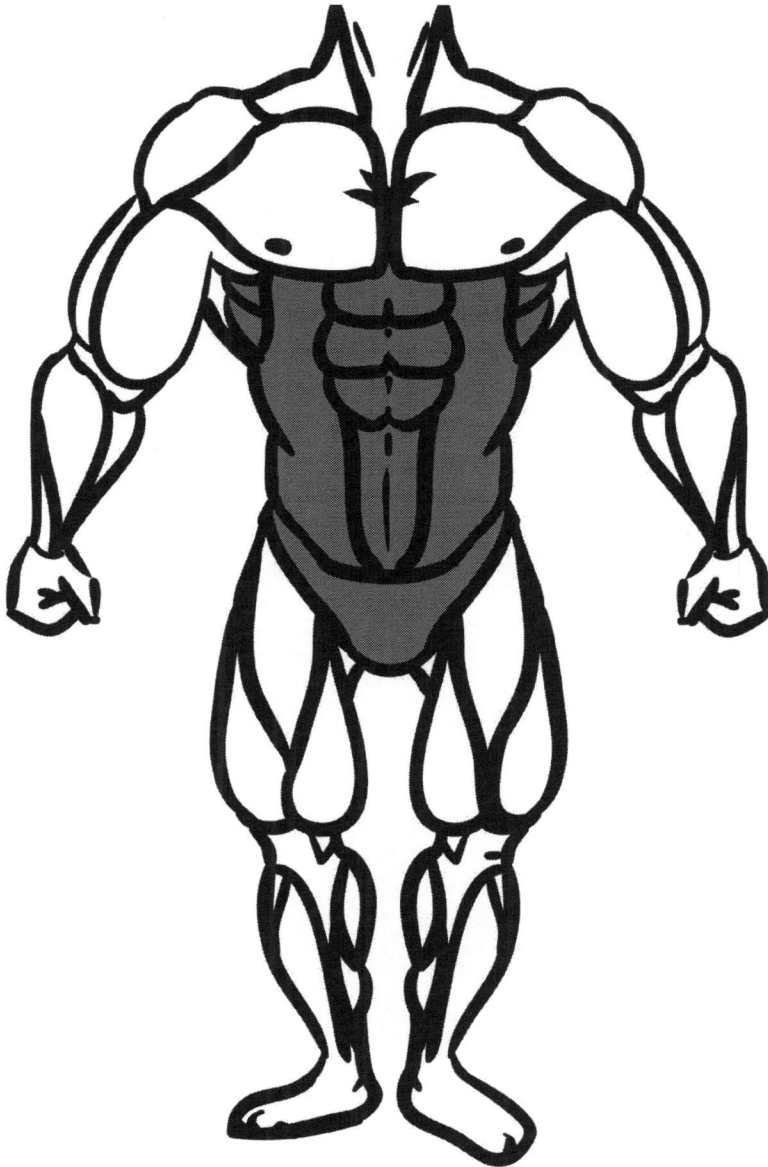

HIP ROTATES

Get your hula on to open up those hip flexors and increase your range of motion.

Perform: 2 sets of 8 repetitions in each direction.

1. Stand upright and place one hand on each hip.

2. Slowly rotate your hips clockwise in a 'hula' movement, aiming to keep your knees and back neutral, focusing the movement in your hips.

3. Repeat the movement counter-clockwise.

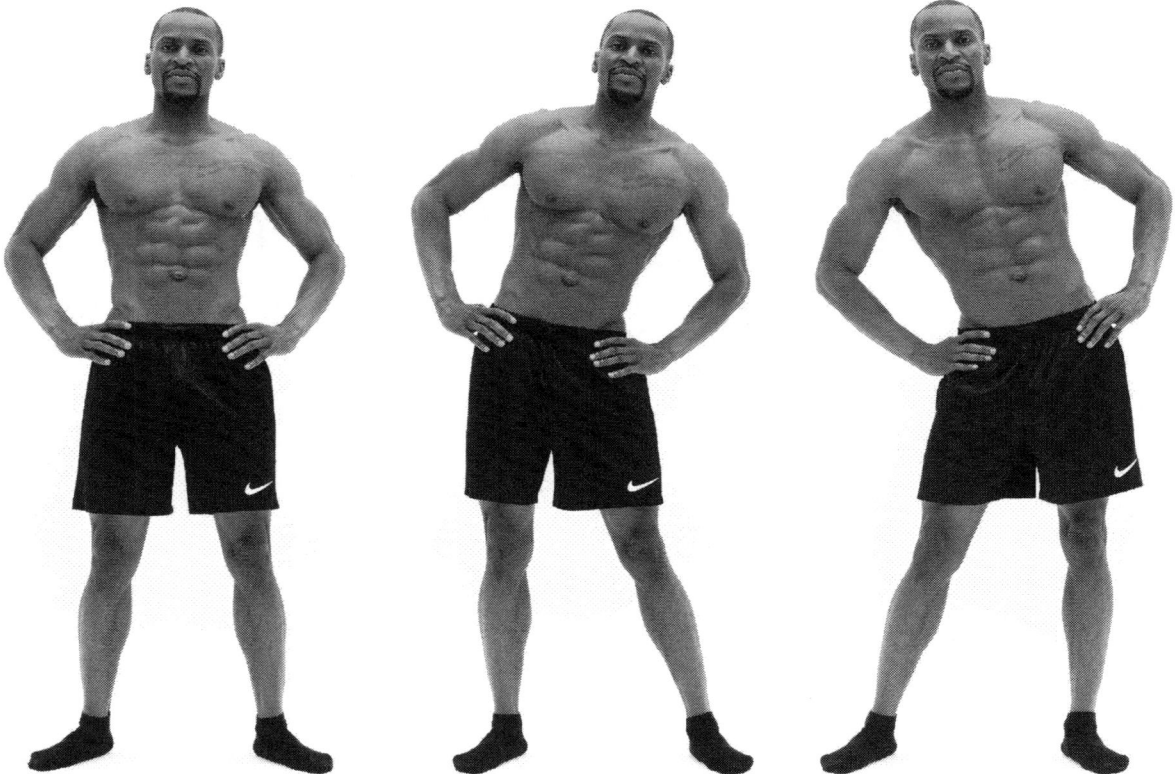

SIDE LEANS

Tight obliques and an inflexible lower spine can greatly inhibit your range of motion, so perform this movement to loosen up these areas.

Perform: 5 repetitions in each direction.

You will need: a long, lightweight bar.

1. Stand upright with your feet just wider than shoulder width apart, grasping the bar over your head.

2. Keeping your arms straight, feet rooted and shoulders in position, lean over to one side to stretch out the other.

3. When you have reached as low as possible, reverse the movement and repeat the exercise on the other side of your body.

Variation: You can perform this exercise without a bar if needs be, simply lean over to one side and grab your leg with the closest hand, bringing the other arm up overhead.

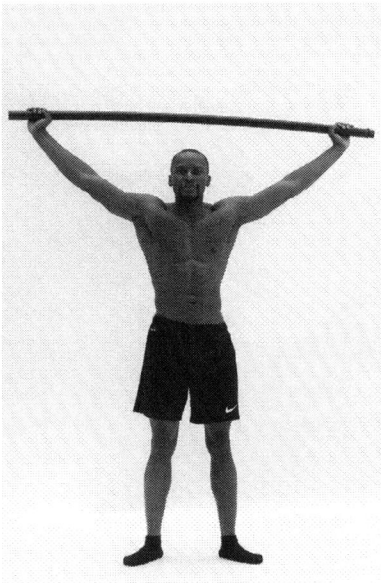

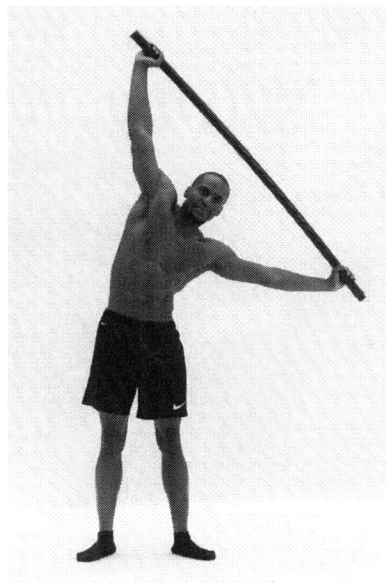

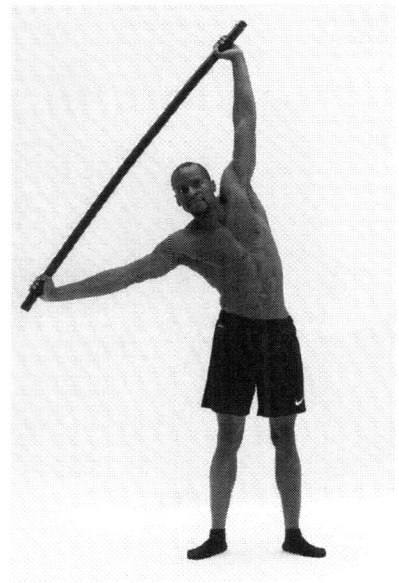

LOWER BODY

Even if you're not stretching your lower body you will still be using it to get around so it's good practice to perform these exercises, too. Check out the following and incorporate them into your routine, or simply practice them on off days.

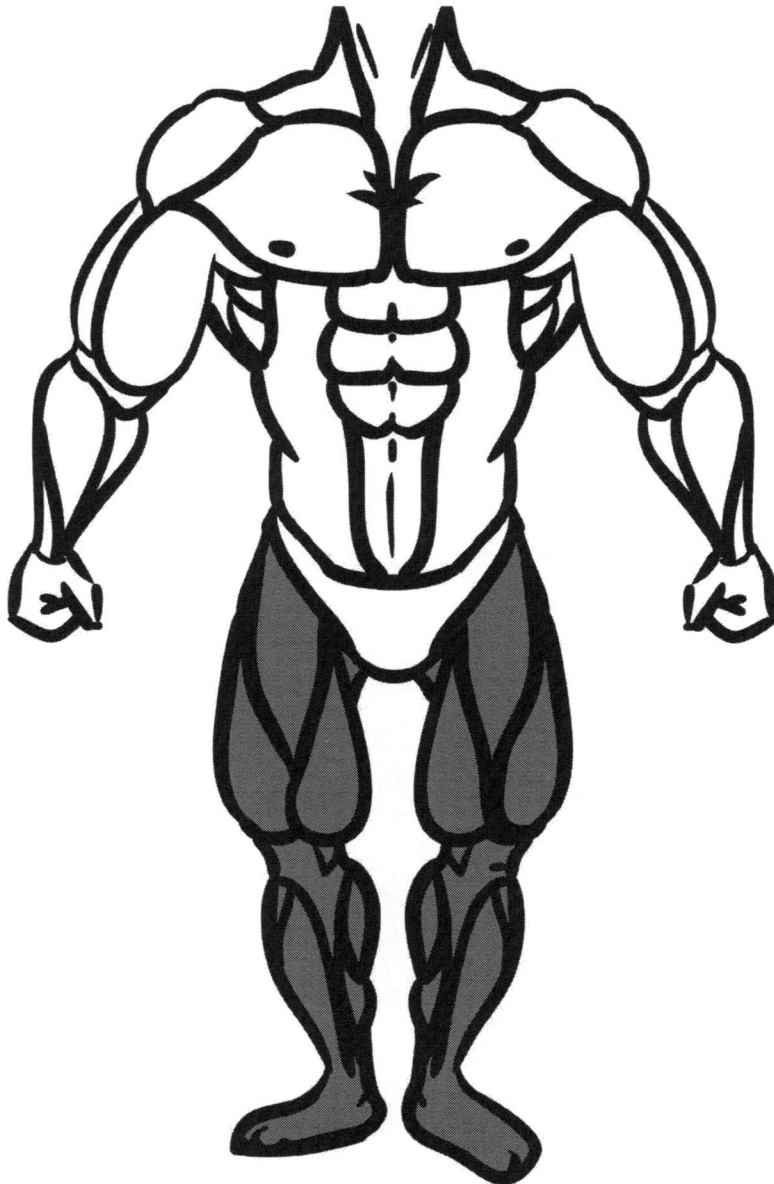

OPEN / CLOSE GATES

This is a staple mobility exercise for elite athletes across a whole range of sports, so it is well worth adding into your routine.

Perform: 8-10 repetitions on each leg.

1. Stand upright and raise one leg upwards, knee bent at 90 degrees.

2. Bring the leg out to the side to open up your hips and groin.

3. Perform the same movement in reverse, first bringing the leg up to the side, then around to the front and back down to the ground.

Variation: You can also perform this exercise on your hands and knees, lifting one knee off the ground, extending it backwards and then bringing it all the way back round the front, and vice versa.

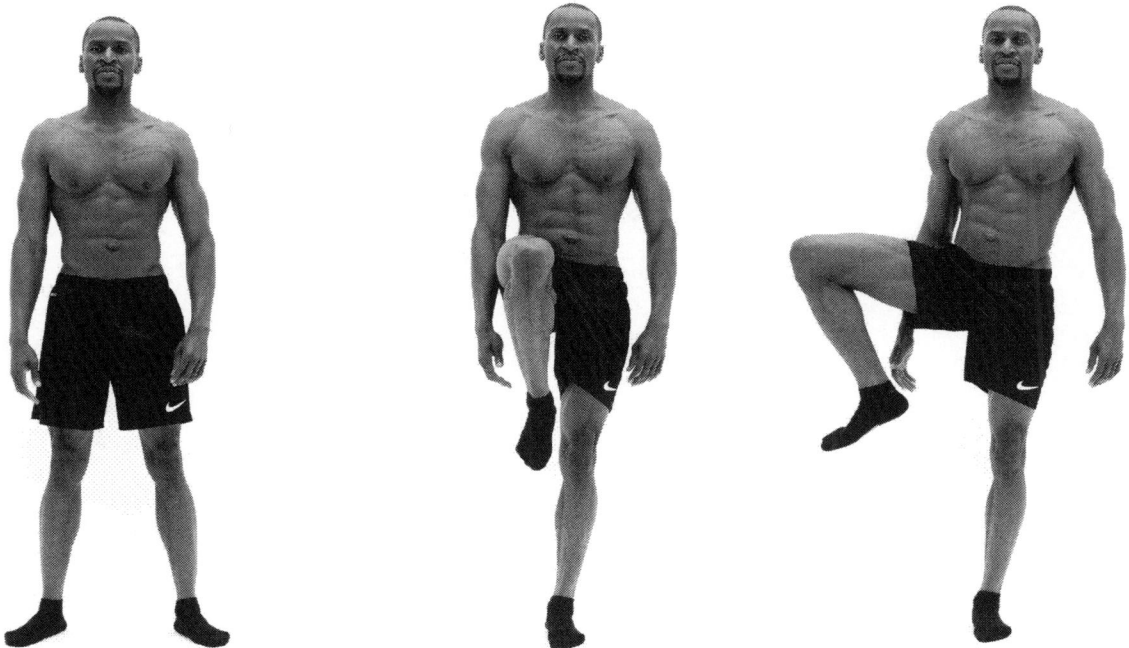

MOUNTAIN CLIMBERS

This is a fantastic, and dynamic, movement to warm up your body and get the blood flowing. Keep your reps unbroken and really lean into the movement to achieve the maximum benefit and increase your hip mobility.

Perform: 8 reps.

1. Assume the push-up position with your arms completely locked out, bringing your left leg forward and placing your foot beside your left hand.

2. Push both feet off the ground and quickly switch them. Now your right foot should be forward and your left out back. This counts as one rep.

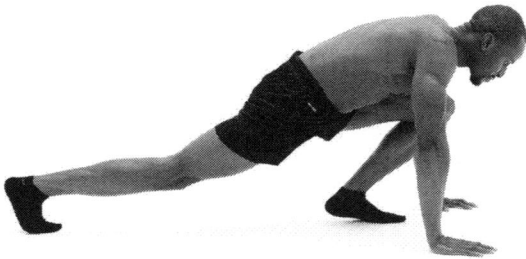

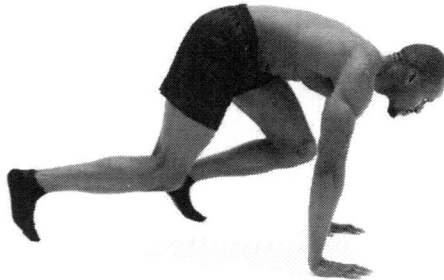

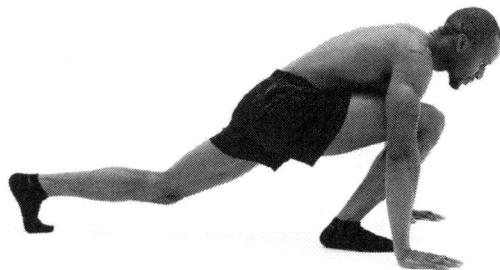

FROG HOPS

This is another excellent exercise to improve your hip mobility, and prepare your body for any exercise involving the lower body.

Perform: 8 reps.

1. Assume the push-up position with arms fully locked out.

2. Leave your hands in place, and jump forward with your feet, landing with them just outside your hands.

3. Reverse the movement and return to the start to complete one rep.

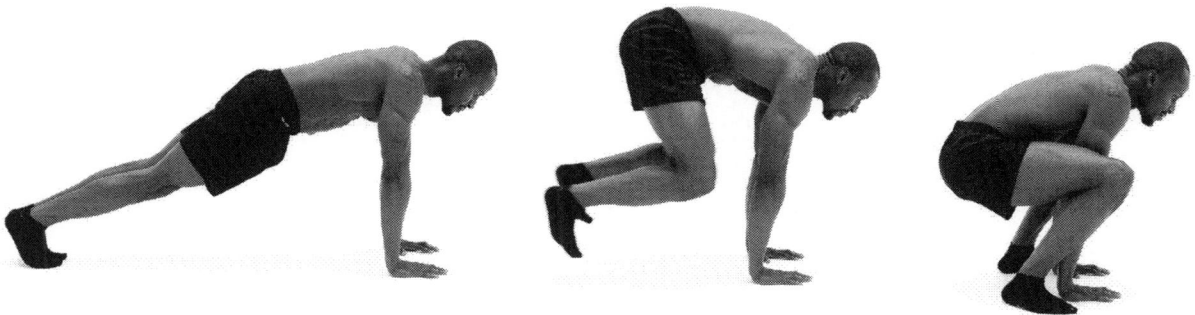

12. KEY STRETCHES

We have arrived! You will find a selection of key stretches in the coming pages, designed to target commonly tight muscles. This is not a set stretching program, and hold times are just a suggestion to get started. You'll find some tips on building your own schedule in the next chapter. Remember to revisit and apply the techniques you have learned.

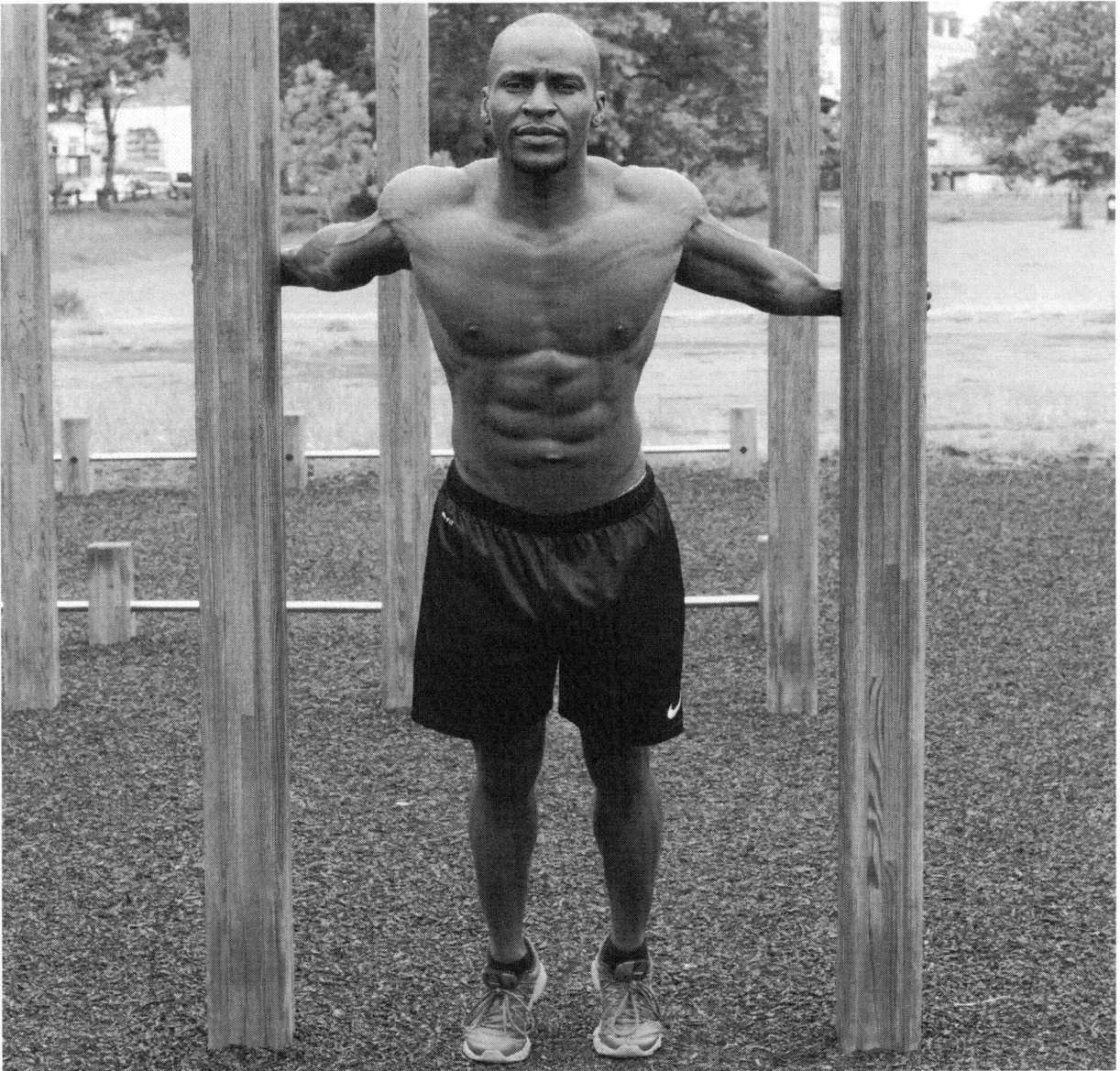

UPPER BODY

The upper body takes a beating during calisthenics training, so be sure to stretch after each session. By improving your flexibility you will also get more out of your workouts, therefore enjoying greater results. We'll start from the top and work our way down.

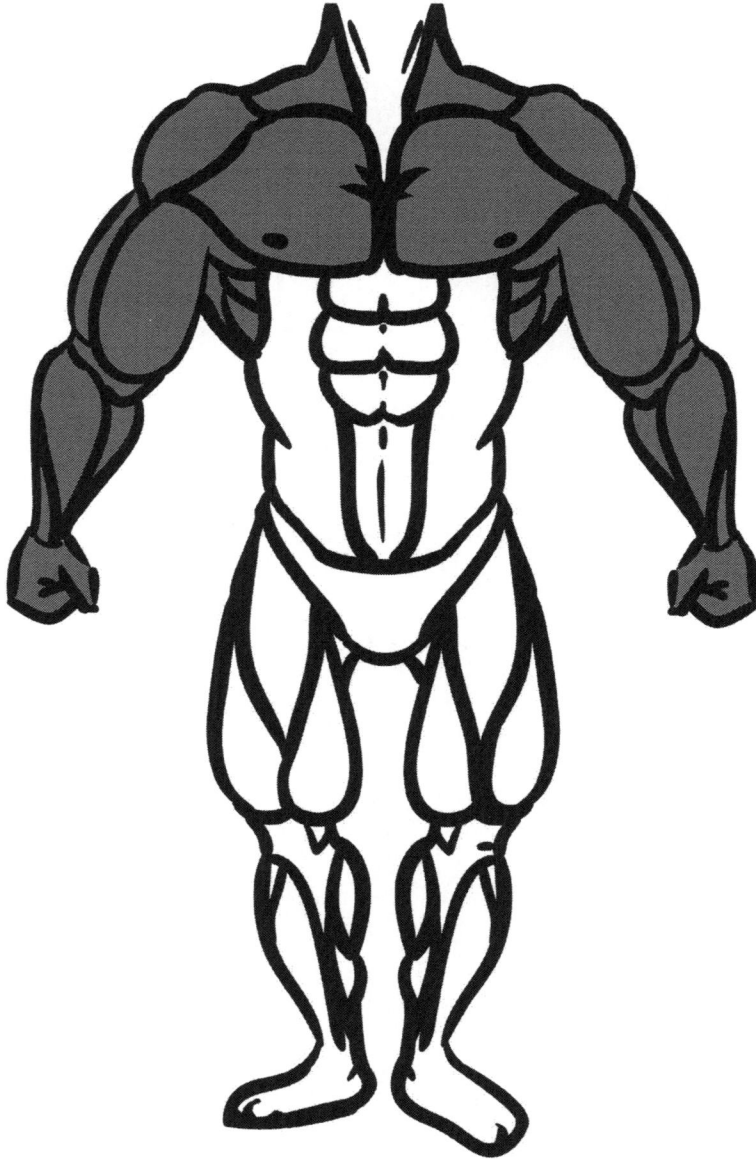

WRISTS & FOREARMS

Great as preparation for handstands as well as all-round strength, get to know both these variations to strengthen your wrists.

Perform: 10-20 second holds per side.

1. Get on your knees and place your palms flat, fingers facing forward, just in front of your knees. Be gentle with this stretch!

2. Lock your arms and slowly lean forwards as far as you can without raising your palms, and hold for the allotted time.

3. Return to start position and repeat the exercise, this time with your fingers facing towards you and leaning backwards instead of forwards.

Variation: If you find this too difficult then use a wall to perform a similar stretch.

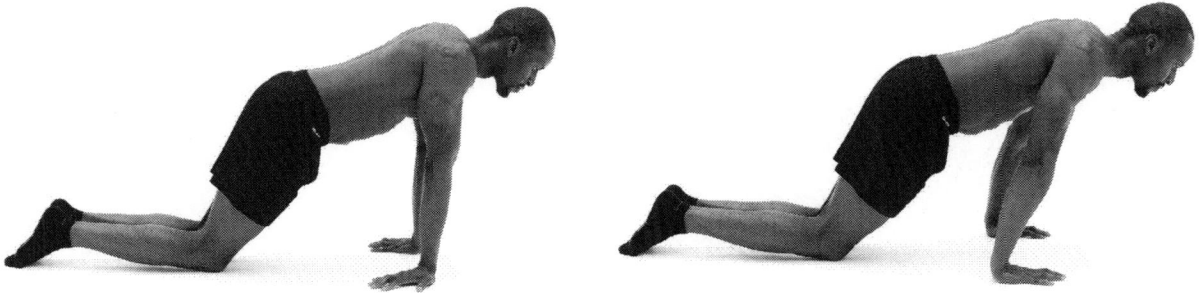

CHEST & SHOULDERS

This stretch is essential in opening up two of the largest muscle groups in your upper body. Find somewhere comfortable and relax into it.

Perform: 15-30 second holds.

1. Get onto your hands and knees, then stretch your arms out in front of you.

2. With your hands and knees rooted to the spot, bring your chest down towards the ground, exhaling as you go. Remember to hold and repeat until you reach your limit.

3. When your chest and shoulders are as low as possible, reset. Place your arms on a high platform to increase the shoulder stretch.

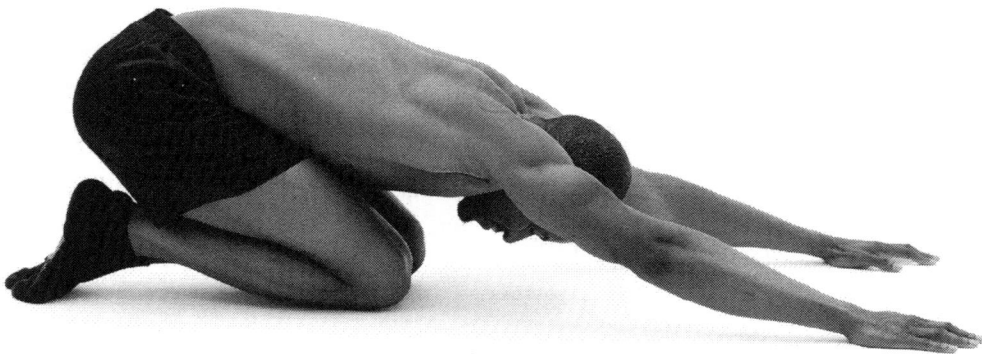

CHEST II

Your chest bears the brunt of almost every upper body exercise in calisthenics, so keep it properly conditioned with this simple stretch.

Perform: 10-30 second holds.

You will need: upright parallel bars or door frame.

1. Stand between the bars or door frame and stretch your arms out to the sides, placing your palms flat on the surface.

2. Ensuring your arms stay straight, lean forward and stretch out your chest, holding for the allotted time. Use the techniques you have learned to gradually increase, then reset.

Variations:

• If you don't have parallel bars use a single bar to stretch one side at a time. Instead of leaning forward, simply turn your body away from your affixed hand to stretch out one side of your chest then repeat on the other.

• You can also perform this exercise on a flat surface, rooting one hand against it and rotating away from that hand.

• Place a medicine ball or other platform on the floor and kneel beside it. Place one arm up on the platform, and then lower your body down to stretch out that side of your chest.

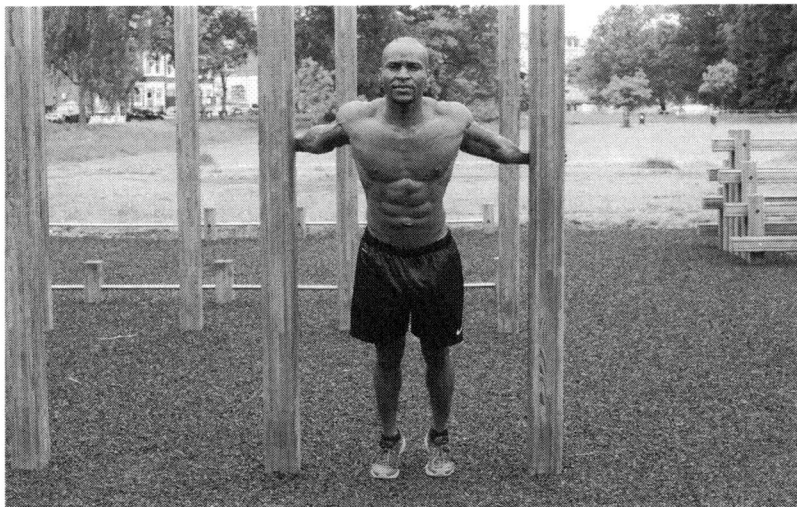

UPPER BACK

This is another area that will take a beating as you condition your body, so get into the habit of stretching it out.

Perform: 10-30 second holds.

You will need: a study bar or fixture.

1. Grab a straight bar or other immovable fixture with one hand.

2. Keeping your arm locked, slowly lean back to stretch out your lattisumus dorsi (lat) on that side.

3. Bring your free arm around in front of your body to stretch further and hold for the allotted time. Repeat on the other side for an effective back stretch.

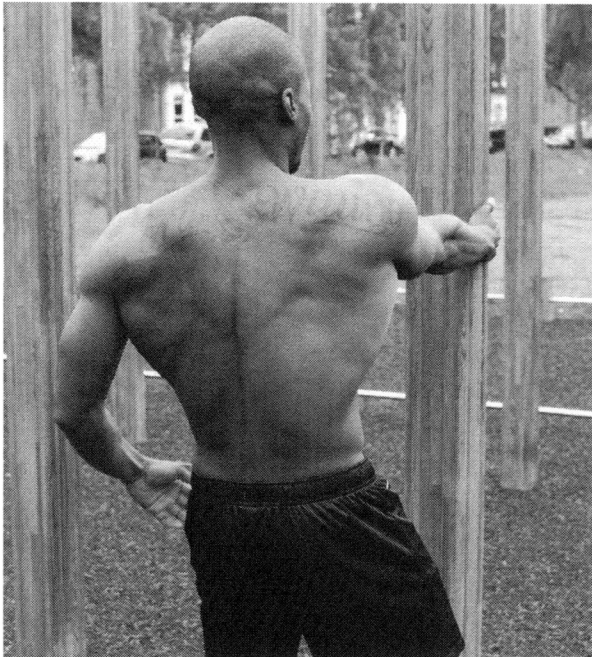

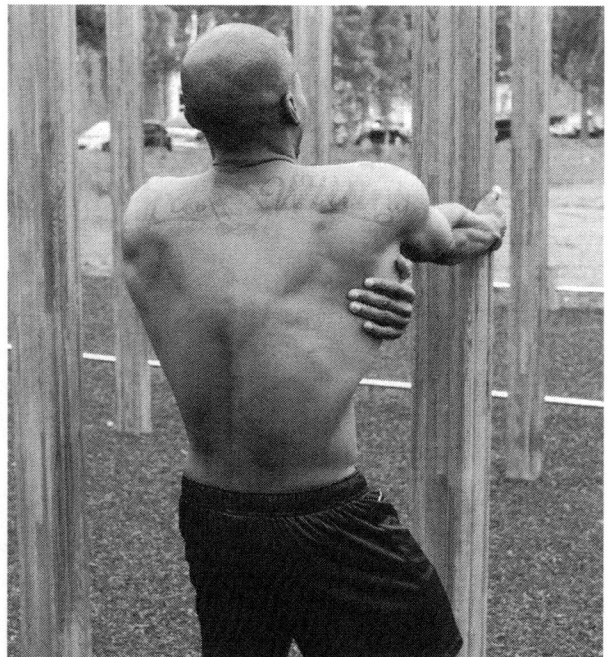

CORE

Everyone covets a chiseled core, and combining mobility and flexibility exercises with bodyweight training will help you achieve just that. You'll find this part quick and easy.

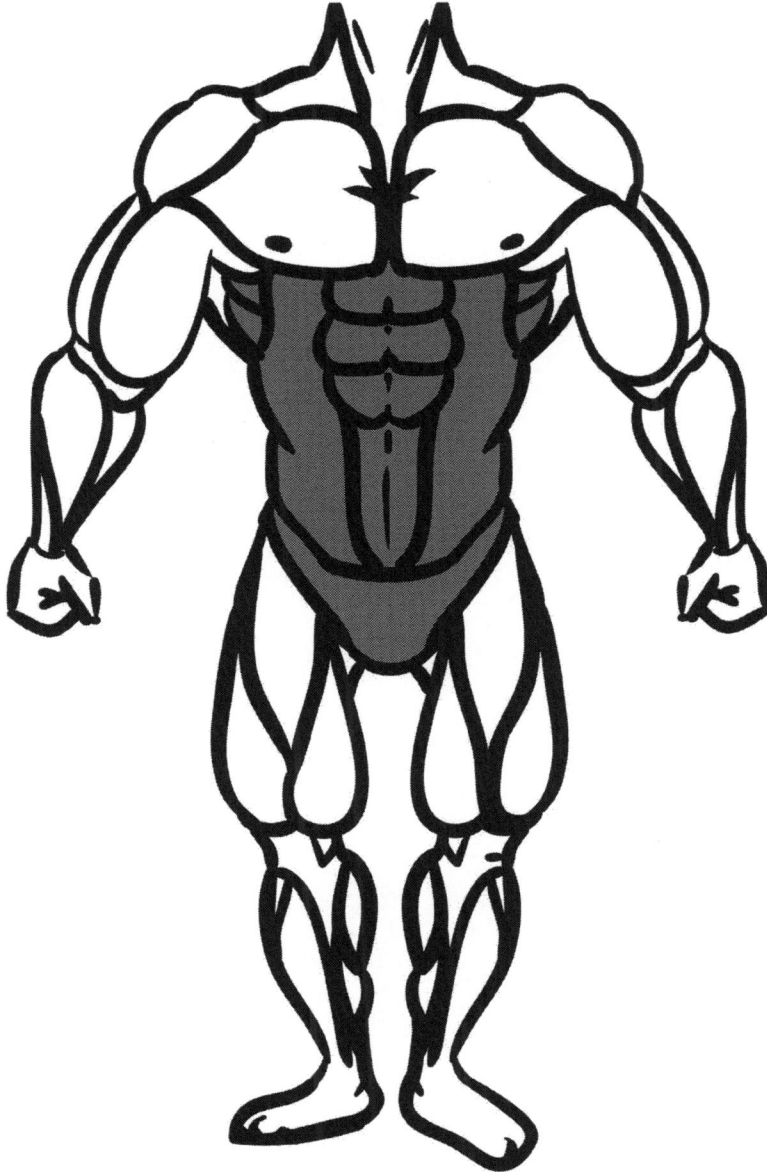

SIDE STRETCH

Prepare your lats, obliques, and lower back for movement with this standing side stretch, the same movement covered in mobility previously. As with all stretches, you don't want to be straining against the movement. Instead, let your muscles relax and fall into the stretch for maximum benefit.

Perform: 5 second holds per side.

You will need: a long, lightweight bar.

1. Stand upright with your feet just wider than shoulder-width apart, grasping the bar over your head.

2. Keeping your arms straight, feet rooted and shoulders in position, lean over to one side to stretch out the other. Imagine glass walls in front and behind you, do not twist!

3. When you have reached as low as possible, reverse the movement and repeat the exercise on the other side of your body.

Variation: You can perform this exercise without a bar if needs be, simply lean over to one side and grab your leg with the closest hand, bringing the other arm up overhead.

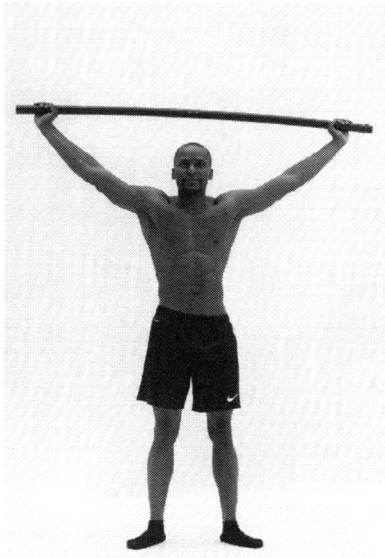

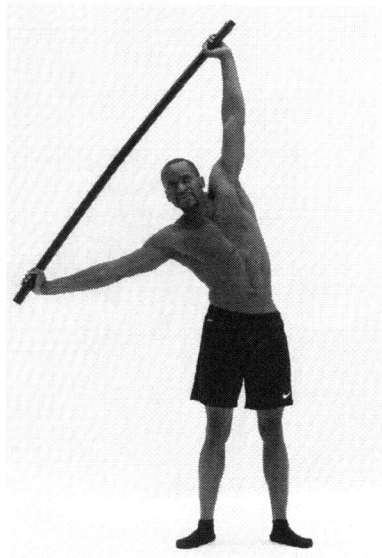

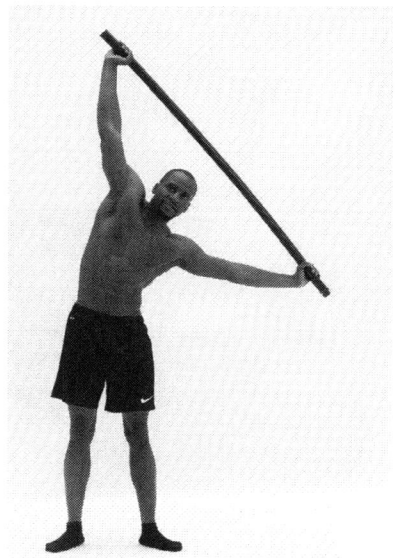

COBRA

If you've ever done yoga you'll know this one as the 'cobra' already. For everyone else, here it is, ideal for opening up your lower back and hips.

Perform: 15-30 second hold time.

1. Lie on your stomach and place your palms flat on the floor, similar to a standard push-up position, fingers facing forward, about shoulder-width apart.

2. With your hips rooted to the ground, raise your head and look upwards, allowing your spine to arch and hold for allotted time.

Variation: If you find this tough to hold, practice raising up onto your forearms and holding the stretch there first.

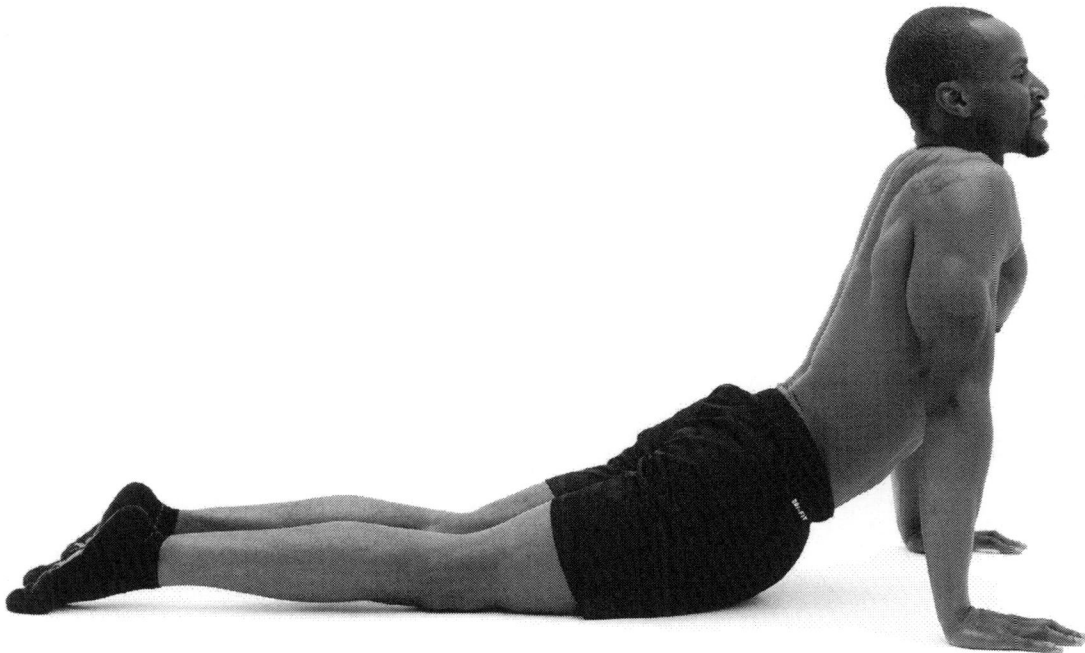

CAT

Another yoga stretch named 'cat', essentially designed to stretch the opposite way to cobra, opening up your back nicely.

Perform: 5-10 second hold time.

1. Get on your hands and knees, palms flat directly underneath your shoulders, fingers facing forward.

2. Drop your head and arch your back as if trying to look at your naval, and hold for the allotted amount of time.

Variation: To turn this into a mobility exercises, get into position and then transition to a downwardly arched back, raising your head up. Moving between the two in a fluid motion is a great way to warm up.

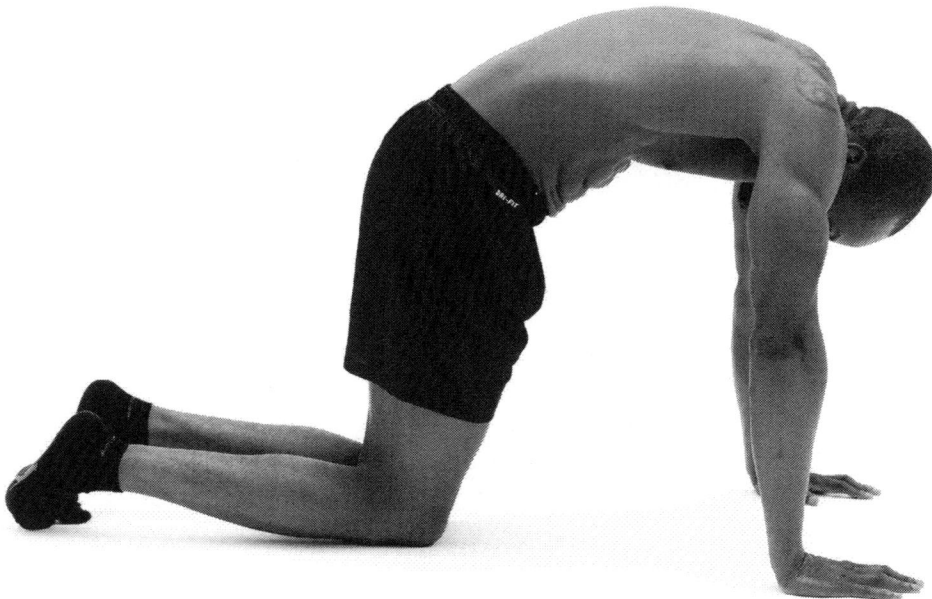

LOWER BODY

Last but by no means least is lower body flexibility. Not only will this help you achieve your dream body, it will also prove useful in everyday life, especially as the years go by. Don't let tight hamstrings, hip flexors or other problem areas hold you back. Let's go!

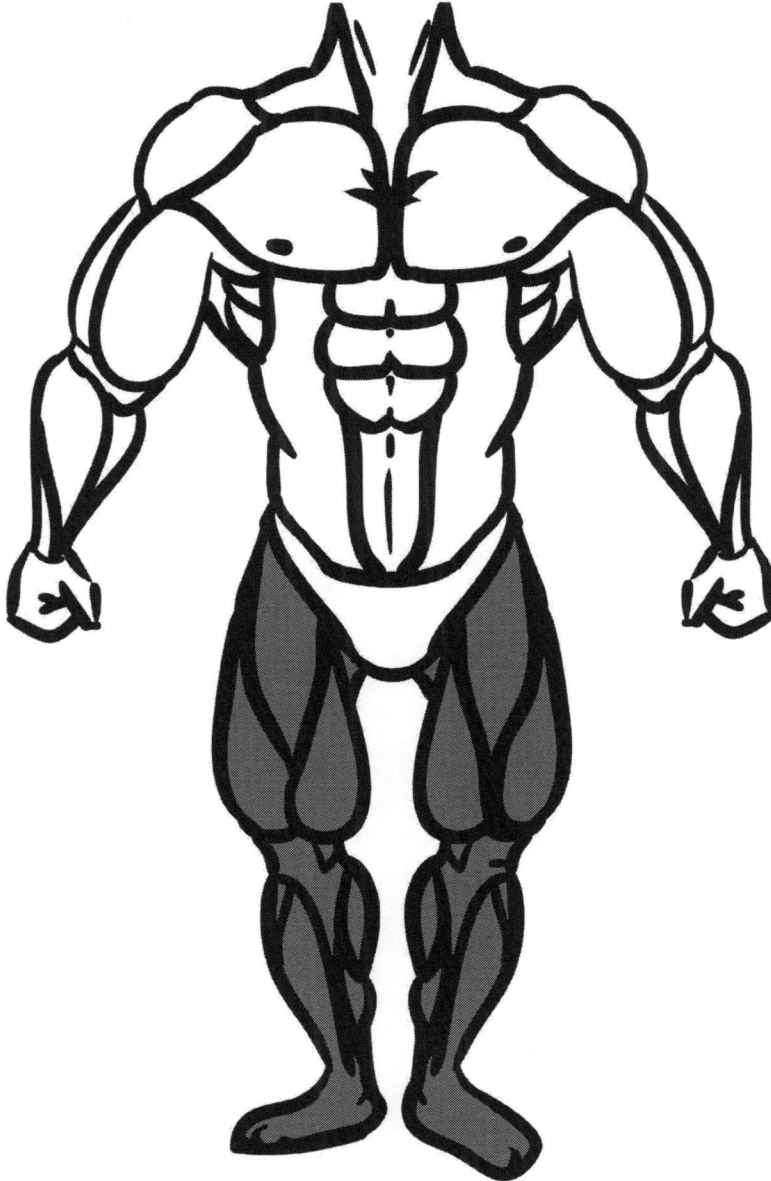

CALVES

Essential for strength and stability, you must ensure your calves are flexible enough to cope with the demands of calisthenics. And, of course, for showing off at barbecues!

Perform: 30 seconds hold time for each leg.

1. Get into push-up position.

2. Take one foot and rest the top of it on the heel of the other.

3. Slowly push the heel of the standing foot down as far as possible and hold for allotted time. You can also perform this exercise standing and pushing against a wall.

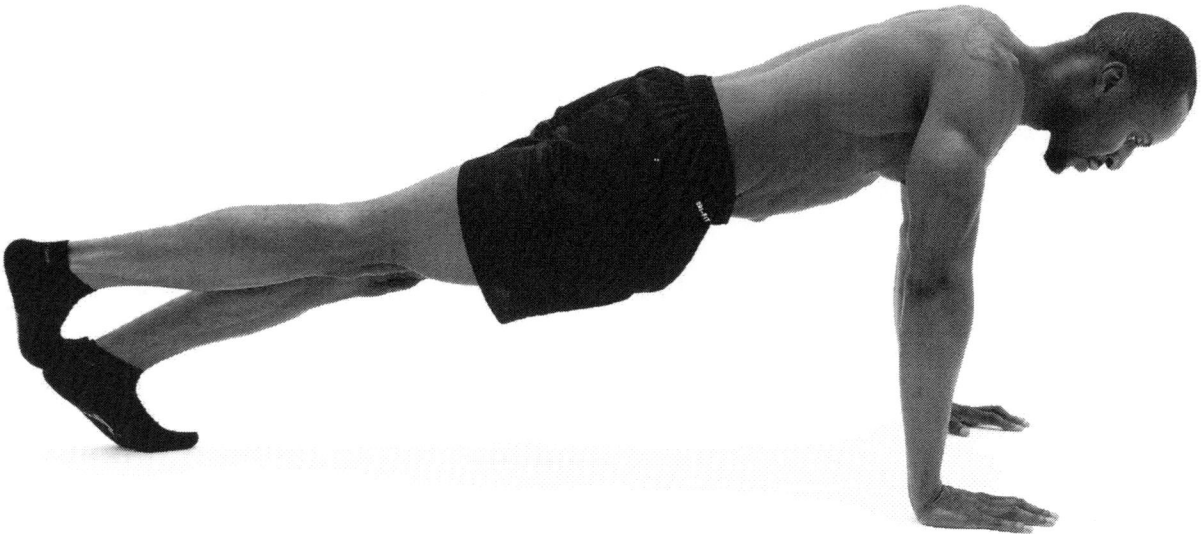

HAMSTRINGS

Most people have tight hamstrings, which can severely inhibit your range of lower body motion. Loosen them up like so:

Perform: 30 second hold time on each leg.

1. Sit down with both legs stretched out in front of you, toes pointing upwards.

2. Bring one foot towards you so the sole is against the inner thigh of the other leg.

3. Keeping your back straight, lean forwards towards the toes of your outstretched leg and hold for allotted time.

To get a back stretch, try to 'fold' your body over and reach forward as below. Don't confuse the two stretches, and make sure you are feeling it in the proper place.

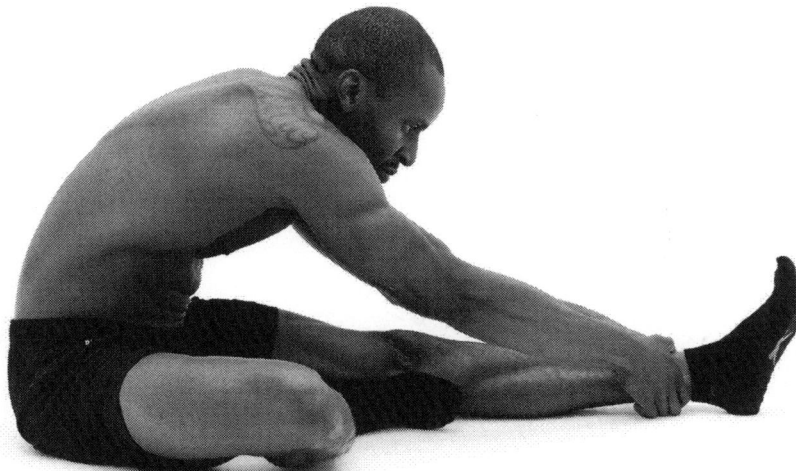

GROIN

Opening up your groin will also open up your hips. You are probably beginning to see how everything is linked together now, so you should never neglect one area in favor of another.

Perform: 15-30 second hold time.

1. Sit down and bring the soles of your feet together.

2. Keeping your back straight, pull your feet towards your body as close as possible.

3. Try to move your knees outwards to touch the floor. If you cannot do this with leg power alone, use your elbows or hands for a little assistance.

4. Hold for allotted time. You may find one side tighter than the other here, but don't worry, it will even out over time.

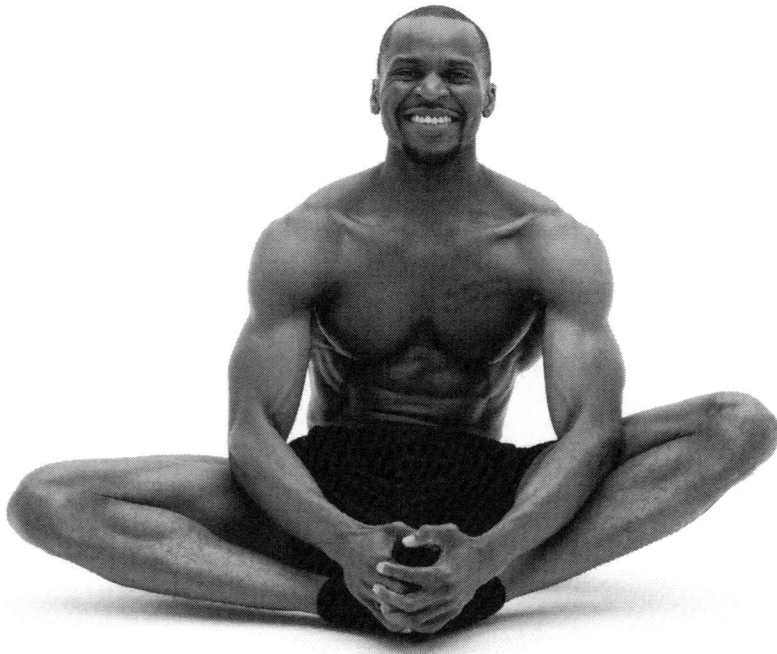

GLUTES

This is a hugely powerful part of your body, driving some of the most important motions required for lower body activities, which is why professional athletes and sports stars often have backsides like Beyoncé.

Perform: 15-30 second hold time on each side.

1. Lay on your back.

2. Bend the knee of one leg and bring it towards you, grasping the leg underneath your hamstring area with both hands.

3. Bring the other leg up and over so the ankle is resting just above the knee of the leg you are holding.

4. Pull the leg you are holding towards you to create a stretch in the opposite side and hold for allotted time.

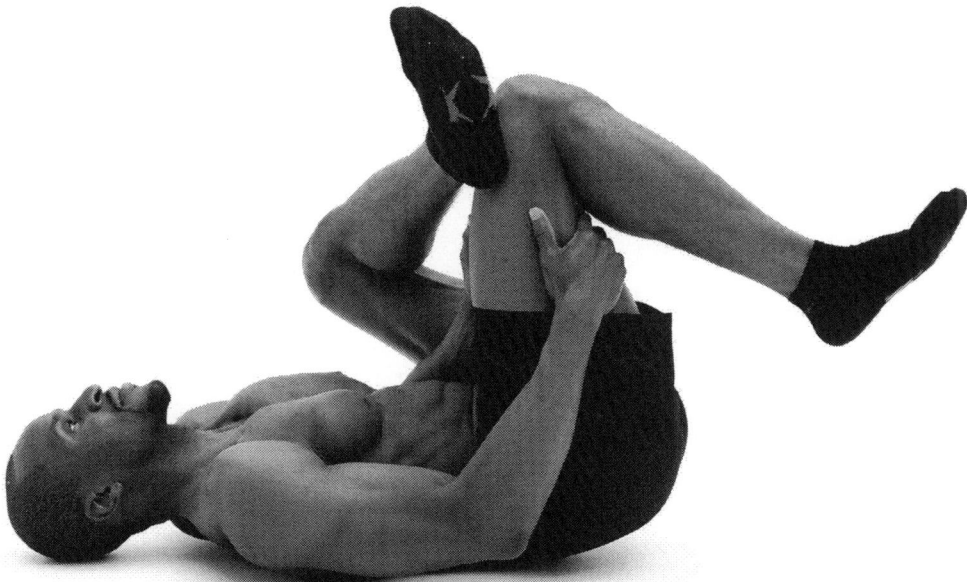

HIP FLEXOR

Your hip flexors work in harmony with your glutes so you can't stretch one without the other. Check this out:

Perform: 15-30 second hold time on each side

1. Stand upright, then place one foot forward.

2. Bend the knee of your front foot and, keeping your body straight and rear foot on the spot, lean forward.

3. When you feel a stretch in the top of your back leg, hold for allotted time.

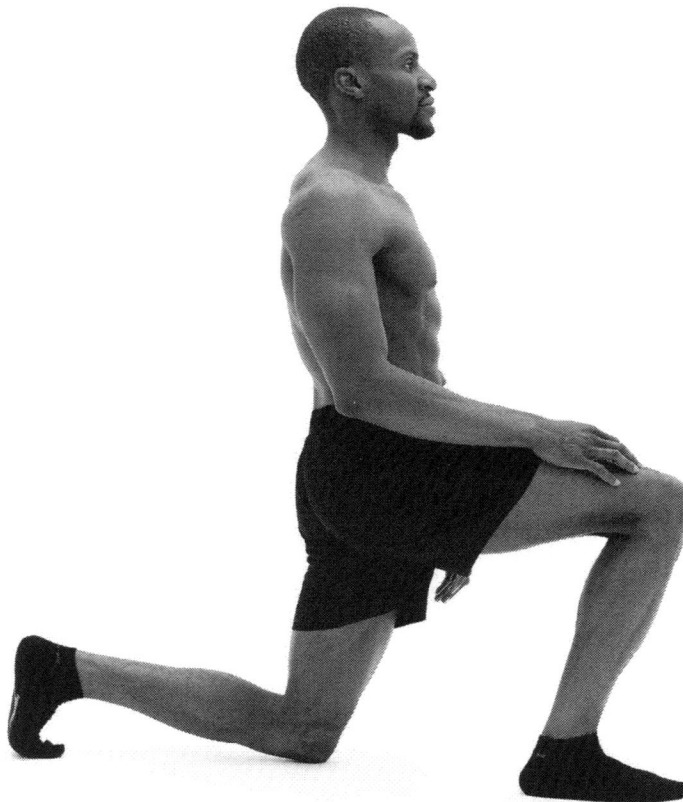

HIPS II

Here, we'll focus on your hips, groin, and hammies, areas that are chronically tight in many people.

Perform: 15-30 second hold.

1. Start at a comfortable sitting position on the floor, and then spread your legs, pushing outward from the hips.

2. Slowly lean forward as far as possible into the space between your legs, and hold for allotted time. Try to maintain a straight back here.

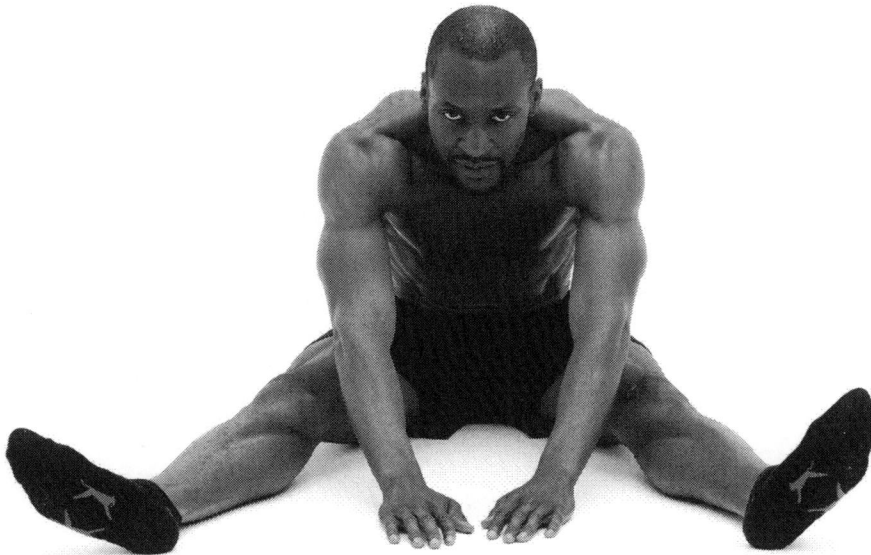

DEEP SQUAT

The squat is an exercise in itself, but we can make it – and almost every other lower body exercise – more effective by practicing the deep squat routinely. Because this one takes a little longer than the others you may prefer to do it on off days or after a heavy lower body session.

Perform: 3-5 minutes or more hold time in each session.

1. Stand with your feet just beyond shoulder width apart, toes pointing out slightly at a comfortable, neutral angle.

2. Bend your knees and lower down into a squat position, ensuring you keep your lower back straight and push your hips back while doing so.

3. Once in position, clasp your hands together and rest your elbows just inside your knees, creating leverage to push your legs outward slightly.

4. Hold for 5 minutes, or as long as you can comfortably.

Variation: If you struggle to maintain your balance at first, place your legs either side of a sturdy pole or fixture and hold onto that to ensure you maintain the proper form.

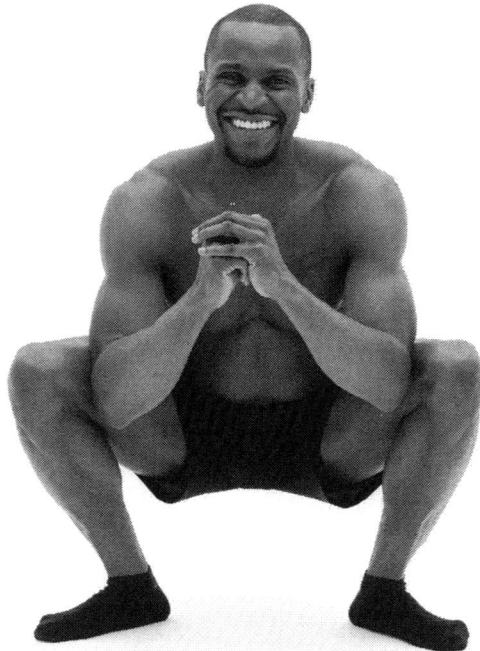

QUADRICEPS

Another massive muscle group vitally important to both calisthenics and day-to-day life are your quads. Keep them happy with this simple stretch:

Perform: 15-30 second hold time.

1. Lie down flat on your stomach.

2. Bend one knee and bring the foot towards your glutes.

3. Grasp the foot with your hand and pull it towards your glutes, then hold for allotted time. Make sure you can feel it in your quads and not in your knee ligaments.

That covers the essential stretching for major muscle groups. Remember to stretch after each workout to aid recovery and increase range of motion and, subsequently, strength.

Listen to your body and seek advice from a specialist if you are unsure about anything. You should be using this advice as a general guideline to help build your own stretching routine rather than sticking to it exactly as it's written above.

For a comprehensive guide on building superhuman strength through flexibility, pick up our companion book on Amazon. Just search 'Pure Calisthenics Flexibility'.

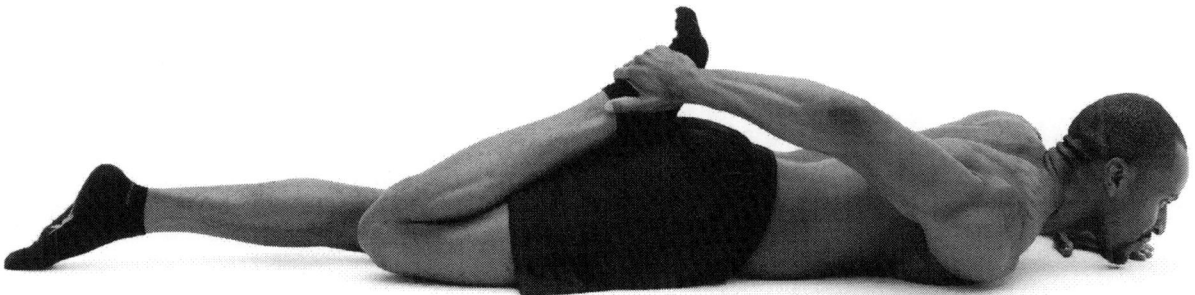

13. STRETCHING PROGRAM

Stretching schedules, just like workout programs, are best designed to suit individual needs. For example, some folk may have very tight hamstrings from years of playing soccer or other sports which require explosive movements, while others may have poor range of motion in the shoulders as a result of hunching over a desk at work.

For this reason there is no 'one size fits all' approach to stretching schedules. Instead, you are encouraged to work with a professional to design one or, if you have plenty of experience designing programs and feel confident in your level of knowledge, work with the below tips to put together your own routine.

DAYS PER WEEK

Depending on your schedule and personal goals, anywhere between 2-4 days a week is normally sufficient. Start out easy and work your way up. Your body will let you know if you are taxing it too much, and you will soon work out your sweet spot.

SETS AND REPS

Think of this just like sets and reps for any other form of exercise. Most people perform between 2-5 sets per exercise, and that is the same general guideline here, too.

Once again, start out at the lower end of the scale and see how your body responds. Most folk will find 2-3 sets per stretch sufficient. If your feel particularly sore the day after stretching that is a sure sign that you are doing too many days or too many sets, so keep tweaking until you find your groove.

PROGRESSION

I've you've ever lifted weights you'll probably be familiar with basic progression during sets, i.e. the act of adding a little more weight each time. The same concept can apply to stretching, too. If you feel confident and capable, try to push yourself a little bit more as you progress through each set. After all, we are not just trying to reach our thresholds here, but redefine them.

TIMING

If you already have a workout plan in place, try to incorporate your stretching regime into it. You should already be stretching after each workout anyway, but you can now take it beyond a simple cool-down and use this time to reinvent your range of motion and compound your strength gains. Get serious about stretching, make time for it and you will be rewarded with mind-blowing results.

You should not need to perform a full stretching routine before each workout, but you absolutely must be warming up. The key is to know the difference between the two. Generally speaking, pre-workout warm-ups should begin with mobility and motion work. Any stretches incorporated here should be used simply to limber up a specific area prior to an exercise. You needn't be doing full body drills before every session.

First thing in the morning is not a good time to stretch your back due to the changes that can occur in the spine overnight. You should also avoid performing your full stretching routine before bedtime.

CREATING A PROGRAM

If you are confident enough to create your own program - by which we mean you should have complete knowledge of every major muscle group, fully understand the concepts contained in this guide and also have extensive experience with stretching and exercise - then the 3 x 3 is a good place to start.

This is a simple schedule consisting of 3 days per week, 3 sets per exercise. But which exercises? That, of course, depends on your personal goals. This is where a consultation with a professional can be invaluable because, in just a few short minutes, they will be able to identify your weakest links and advise on a regime to strengthen them.

In the absence of that, however, the most commonly compromised areas are the hip flexors and hamstrings. This is largely down to an increasingly sedentary lifestyle. Being seated, for example, shortens the hip flexors and, as we know, your nervous system becomes accustomed to that setting over time.

Hamstrings can also be a victim of this effect or, on the flip side, can become tight due to overuse or injury. Either way, you are likely to have the most room for improvement within these areas.

Continuing the lower body theme, glutes, quads and calves are other muscles to target, while in the core area your lower back and obliques can benefit from stretching.

The upper body tends not to be as big an issue, but poor posture, muscle imbalances and overuse or injury can also contribute to problems here. The most common issues here are tight shoulders, being drawn towards your chest as a result of being hunched over at a desk. Fixing your postural problems and changing up your work environment to include, for example, a standing or treadmill desk, are just as important here as a proper stretching and mobility regime.

The upper back tends not to be too tight, since it is actually used to overextending as a result of the shoulders being hunched forward, however the lats can often benefit from opening up. Aside from this, good wrist and arm stretches will be very beneficial when it comes to mastering the more demanding moves that intermediate to advanced calisthenics has to offer.

We recommend identifying your key problem areas and then prioritizing those in your program. This will almost always include the hip flexors, and likely hamstrings too. Get into the habit of stretching these consistently, and then add in other muscles to the mix.

The stretches shown in chapter 14 cover some of the most common areas, so take a look, try them out and see if you can spot your weak links.

Consistency

Consistency is the key to progress. You must be just as committed to your stretching program as your workout routine. Developing flexibility in tandem with strength is the secret to going superhuman, so don't approach this with a half-assed attitude.

Be sure to be consistent with each part of your body, too. For example, recovering from a hamstring strain on one side doesn't mean you should focus all your attention there. If you fail to distribute the workload evenly then you will quickly develop a muscular imbalance, which is a shortcut to even bigger issues than you may have started with.

One of the most effective ways to stick to a stretching schedule is to find someone who can hold you accountable. Ideally that will be a personal trainer or, failing that, simply someone to share your journey on the road to become supple. Just don't feel that you have to compete or out-do each other, this isn't a competitive sport!

Finally, it helps to have some skin in the game if you want to stay committed. Purchasing a proven program is a powerful financial incentive, as we are all much more likely to take action when we have placed money on the table.

That's about as much advice as we can offer here, but it should be more than enough to get started. If you're new to calisthenics as well as stretching, then read on for a brief introduction to the fastest growing fitness movement in the world!

14. Bonus Chapter: What is Calisthenics?

If you're reading this book then the chances are you've already looked into calisthenics, probably read a few articles and watched some videos of seemingly superhuman feats of strength from famous practitioners.

These guys have it all; traps that reach up to their ears, sculpted shoulders, bulging chests, forearms like Popeye, abs you could grate cheese on and legs that could propel them to the moon. And all without pumping iron? Well, pretty much.

How Does it Work?

Calisthenics, by definition, is a form of exercise that consists of various gross motor movements using your own bodyweight for resistance, normally without equipment or apparatus with the exception of basic items such as a pull-up bar.

This is the art of training your body as it was meant to be trained; not by isolating muscle groups and using man-made machinery which you would never find in the real world but by using the tools you already have. Your body becomes your gym and you work it as nature intended.

What Does it Do?

Calisthenics is the art of strengthening your entire body as a unit; eliminating each weak link in the chain until every fiber of your being is working in harmony to form extraordinary levels of strength.

Training like this achieves results you can use in the real world. Think about it, how often do you need to bicep curl something, or flap cables around over your head? These are all man-made inventions designed to make single muscle groups strong IN THE GYM but as soon as we step outside it becomes irrelevant.

To perform at maximum capacity in other sports or just go about your everyday life as the best possible version of yourself you need to be strong everywhere, not just in certain places.

Calisthenics strengthens every muscle group and every link between those muscle groups. It is the ultimate form of exercise for creating true strength that you can use every day whether it be for regular tasks, sport or just showing off!

WHO IS IT FOR?

The simple answer to this question is...everyone. Practicing the art of calisthenics can help anyone achieve a stronger, fitter, more flexible body.

Whether you are a lean athlete seeking to strengthen your entire body, a 180-pound bodybuilder requiring greater range of motion or just completely new to all forms of exercise you WILL feel the benefits of bodyweight work.

Don't just take our word for it. Professional sports teams and military regiments often utilize calisthenics for its explosive results and practical application. You can use your bodyweight to train any place, any time, making it the benchmark fitness solution across the world. Don't get stuck performing isolated exercises in the gym, practice calisthenics and take your gym with you wherever you go!

If you want to learn more about calisthenics, check out our range of books below!

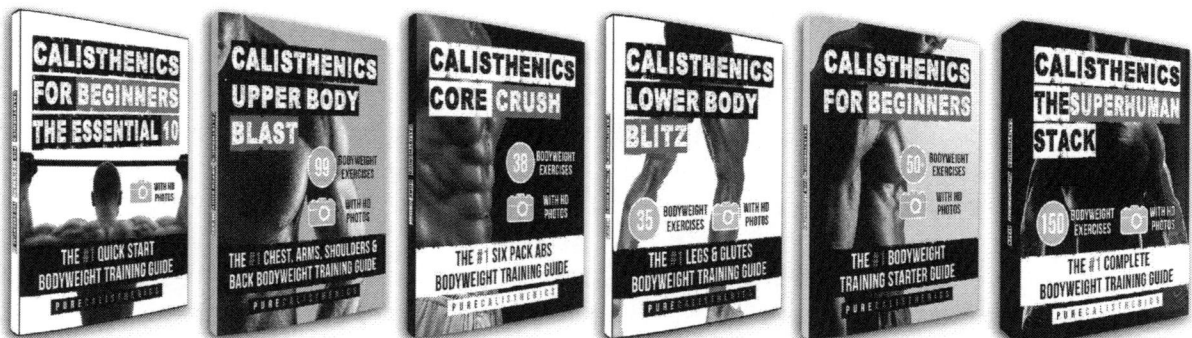

"Have faith in the formula. It will get you there."

Pure Calisthenics

Free Stretching Guide

Don't Forget Yours!

To avoid injury and help accelerate your progress, pick up our free 'Top 10 Stretching Mistakes' guide to make sure YOU aren't falling into these common traps!

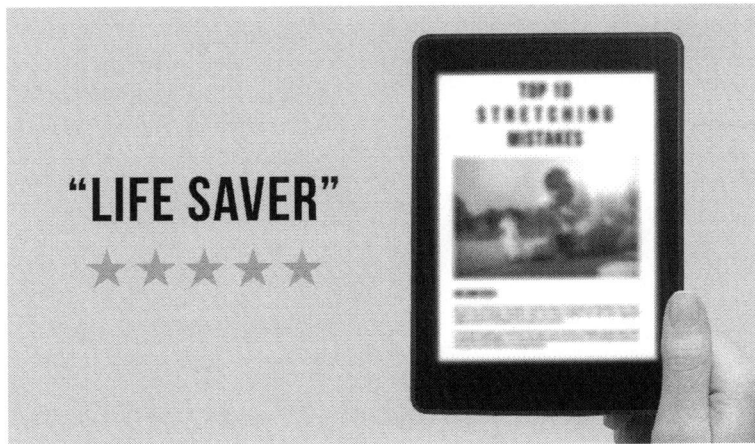

Visit www.purecalisthenics.com/stretching-guide to get it now!

LIKE THIS BOOK?

The calisthenics community is all about sharing ideas and growing together. With that in mind, here's a few ways you can get involved:

1. If you got value from this book, or the free bonus stretching guide, we'd be super stoked if you could head on over to your Amazon purchase history to leave a review. It only takes a few seconds but really helps us keep improving and sharing our stuff :)

2. The most powerful way to boost your progress is to share your journey with a friend. Put a call out on Facebook and Twitter, share this guide with a training partner and go crush it together! Search for us on social media and share your training pics too!

3. To see our other books and resources, search 'Pure Calisthenics' on Amazon and visit www.purecalisthenics.com for bodyweight training tips, equipment reviews, nutrition advice and more.

So, all that remains to say is thanks again for picking up this book. Don't forget to grab your free guide and, as always, train hard!

The Pure Calisthenics Team

Review Now!

Share on Twitter

Share on Facebook

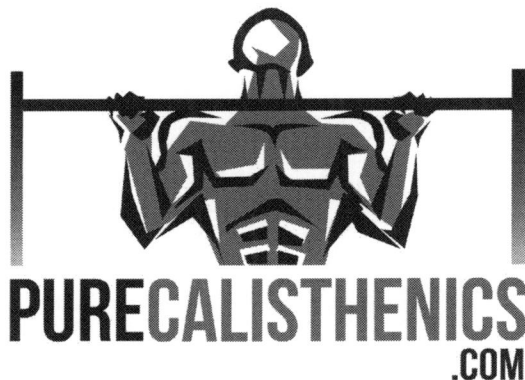

PURECALISTHENICS
.COM

ABOUT THE AUTHORS

In early 2015 a small bunch of dedicated calisthenics practitioners made a decision to share the vast wealth of knowledge they had accumulated about fitness, nutrition, bodyweight exercise and general wellbeing with the rest of the world.

On that day the 'Pure Calisthenics' team was born, and it has since helped spread the movement to all corners of the globe through simple, functional training and tutorials. The guys have had big hits with their books and are consistently helping to bring new people into the game through a steadily growing email and social media community.

The goal of starting the Pure Calisthenics movement was to educate, assist and inspire people regardless of age, gender, training background or end goal. The team is always happiest when diving deep into a project and prefer to spend their days working away in the background to produce high quality, informative tutorials and content.

They guys have a blog over at purecalisthenics.com and are also active on Facebook, Twitter and Instagram, but you will find their best work between the pages of their bestselling books. The SUPERHUMAN Series is transforming lives every single day and the juggernaut shows no sign of slowing down.

By picking up this book you have made the choice to become a person of action and join the Pure Calisthenics community. No matter where you came from, or where you are going, the team will be thrilled to help you get there.

13221729R00061

Printed in Germany
by Amazon Distribution
GmbH, Leipzig